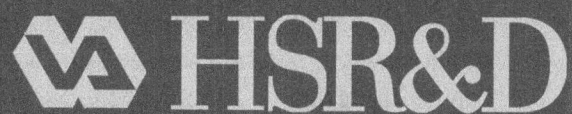

# Rural vs. Urban Ambulatory Health Care: A Systematic Review

May 2011

## Prepared for:

Department of Veterans Affairs
Veterans Health Administration
Health Services Research & Development Service
Washington, DC 20420

## Prepared by:

Evidence-based Synthesis Program (ESP) Center
Minneapolis VA Medical Center
Minneapolis, MN
Timothy J. Wilt, MD, MPH, Director

## Investigators:

Principal Investigator:
Michele Spoont, PhD

Co-Investigators:
Nancy Greer, PhD
Jenny Su, PhD

Research Associates:
Patrick Fitzgerald, MPH
Indulis Rutks, BS

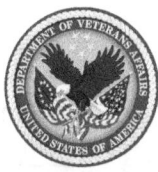

# PREFACE

Health Services Research & Development Service's (HSR&D's) Evidence-based Synthesis Program (ESP) was established to provide timely and accurate syntheses of targeted healthcare topics of particular importance to Veterans Affairs (VA) managers and policymakers, as they work to improve the health and healthcare of Veterans. The ESP disseminates these reports throughout VA.

HSR&D provides funding for four ESP Centers and each Center has an active VA affiliation. The ESP Centers generate evidence syntheses on important clinical practice topics, and these reports help:

- develop clinical policies informed by evidence,

- guide the implementation of effective services to improve patient outcomes and to support VA clinical practice guidelines and performance measures, and

- set the direction for future research to address gaps in clinical knowledge.

In 2009, the ESP Coordinating Center was created to expand the capacity of HSR&D Central Office and the four ESP sites by developing and maintaining program processes. In addition, the Center established a Steering Committee comprised of HSR&D field-based investigators, VA Patient Care Services, Office of Quality and Performance, and Veterans Integrated Service Networks (VISN) Clinical Management Officers. The Steering Committee provides program oversight, guides strategic planning, coordinates dissemination activities, and develops collaborations with VA leadership to identify new ESP topics of importance to Veterans and the VA healthcare system.

Comments on this evidence report are welcome and can be sent to Nicole Floyd, ESP Coordinating Center Program Manager, at nicole.floyd@va.gov.

**Recommended citation:** Spoont M, Greer N, Su J, Fitzgerald P, Rutks I, and Wilt TJ. Rural vs. Urban Ambulatory Health Care: A Systematic Review. VA-ESP Project #09-009;2011.

This report is based on research conducted by the Evidence-based Synthesis Program (ESP) Center located at the Minneapolis VA Medical Center, Minneapolis, MN funded by the Department of Veterans Affairs, Veterans Health Administration, Office of Research and Development, Health Services Research and Development. The findings and conclusions in this document are those of the author(s) who are responsible for its contents; the findings and conclusions do not necessarily represent the views of the Department of Veterans Affairs or the United States government. Therefore, no statement in this article should be construed as an official position of the Department of Veterans Affairs. No investigators have any affiliations or financial involvement (e.g., employment, consultancies, honoraria, stock ownership or options, expert testimony, grants or patents received or pending, or royalties) that conflict with material presented in the report.

# TABLE OF CONTENTS

**EXECUTIVE SUMMARY**

Background.................................................................................................................. 1

Methods .................................................................................................................... 1

Data Synthesis ........................................................................................................... 2

Peer Review ............................................................................................................... 2

Results ....................................................................................................................... 2

Future Research ......................................................................................................... 3

**INTRODUCTION**

Background.................................................................................................................. 5

Definitions of Rurality ................................................................................................ 6

**METHODS**

Topic Development...................................................................................................... 9

Search Strategy .......................................................................................................... 9

Study Selection .......................................................................................................... 10

Data Abstraction ........................................................................................................ 10

Data Synthesis ........................................................................................................... 10

Rating the Body of Evidence...................................................................................... 10

Peer Review............................................................................................................... 11

**RESULTS**

Literature Flow .......................................................................................................... 12

Preventive Care/Ambulatory Care Sensitive Conditions ........................................... 13

Cancer Care ............................................................................................................... 16

Diabetes/End Stage Renal Disease ............................................................................. 20

Cardiovascular Disease .............................................................................................. 23

HIV/AIDS.................................................................................................................. 25

Neurologic Conditions............................................................................................... 26

    Mental Health.................................................................................................. 28

    Processes or Structure of Care ......................................................................... 33

    Use of Medication........................................................................................... 33

    Medical Procedures and Diagnostic Tests........................................................ 35

    Medical Appointments with Providers.............................................................. 35

    Usual Source of Care ....................................................................................... 36

    Provider Availability and Expertise .................................................................. 37

**SUMMARY AND DISCUSSION**

Conclusions and Recommendations............................................................................ 42

Summary of Evidence by Key Question ..................................................................... 42

Research Implications and Recommendations............................................................. 46

**REFERENCES** ....................................................................................................................... 49

**TABLES**

Table 1.    Definitions of Urban and Rural ................................................................................... 7

Table 2.    Explanation of Confidence Scores ............................................................................ 11

Table 3.    Confidence Scores for Preventive Care/Ambulatory Care Sensitive Condition Studies .......... 16

Table 4.    Confidence Scores for Cancer Care Studies .............................................................. 20

Table 5.    Confidence Scores for Diabetes and End-Stage Renal Disease Studies ................... 23

Table 6.    Confidence Scores for Cardiovascular Disease Studies ............................................ 25

Table 7.    Confidence Scores for HIV/AIDS Studies ................................................................ 26

Table 8.    Confidence Scores for Neurologic Conditions Studies ............................................ 28

Table 9.    Confidence Scores for Mental Health Studies .......................................................... 34

Table 10.   Confidence Scores for Processes and Structure of Care Studies .............................. 40

**FIGURES**

Figure 1.   Analytic Framework ................................................................................................... 9

Figure 2.   Flow Diagram of Included Studies ........................................................................... 12

**APPENDIX A.  DATA ABSTRACTION FORM** ........................................................... 58

**APPENDIX B.  PEER REVIEW COMMENTS AND AUTHOR RESPONSES** ................... 59

**APPENDIX C.  EVIDENCE TABLES**

Table 1.    Preventive Care/Ambulatory Care Sensitive Conditions ......................................... 65

Table 2.    Cancer Screening ...................................................................................................... 67

Table 3.    Cancer Care .............................................................................................................. 69

Table 4.    Diabetes/End Stage Renal Disease ........................................................................... 73

Table 5.    Cardiovascular Disease ............................................................................................. 76

Table 6.    HIV/AIDS ................................................................................................................. 78

Table 7.    Neurologic Conditions .............................................................................................. 79

Table 8.    Mental Health ........................................................................................................... 81

Table 9.    Use of Medication ..................................................................................................... 88

Table 10.   Medical Procedures and Diagnostic Tests ............................................................... 90

Table 11.   Medical Appointments with Providers ..................................................................... 91

Table 12.   Usual Source of Care ............................................................................................... 94

Table 13.   Provider Availability and Expertise ......................................................................... 96

# EXECUTIVE SUMMARY

## BACKGROUND

Approximately 3 million veterans, slightly more than one-third of all veterans enrolled in the Department of Veterans Affairs (VA) health care system, live in rural areas. This pattern is likely to continue, as a comparable proportion of Operation Enduring Freedom/Operation Iraqi Freedom (OEF/OIF) veterans are from rural areas. The Rural Veterans Care Act of 2006 was signed into law to improve care for rural veterans. Ensuring that the health care needs of rural veterans are met has become a top priority for VA, resulting in a considerable expansion of community based outpatient clinics (CBOCs), inclusion of rural health/access as a research priority, and creation of the VA Office of Rural Health (ORH) in 2006.

Although there have been reports comparing health quality of life (both physical and mental) for rural and urban veterans, it remains unclear whether the observed lower health quality of life in rural veterans is due to disparities in health care, differences in disease prevalence, or other population differences. This systematic review examines the evidence regarding potential disparities between rural and urban areas in health care provision and delivery, and how differences in health care may contribute to disparities in health outcomes. Differences in rural-urban prevalence rates of diseases and other health conditions are beyond the scope of this review. Because veterans who use VA health care have been found to use more non-VA health care overall, we expanded the focus of this review to include comparisons of rural vs. urban health care in non-VA health systems.

The key questions were:

Key Question #1. Do adults with health care needs who live in rural areas have different intermediate (e.g., hemoglobin A1c [HbA1c], Blood pressure, etc.) or final health outcomes (i.e., mortality, morbidity, quality of life [QOL]) than those living in urban areas?

Key Question #2. Is the structure (e.g., types of available providers) or the process (e.g., likelihood of referral) of health care different for adults with health care needs who live in urban vs. rural environments?

Key Question #3. If there are differences in the structure or the process of health care in rural vs. urban environments, do those differences contribute to variation in overall or intermediate health outcomes for adults with health care needs?

Key Question #4. If there are differences in intermediate or final health outcomes for adult patients with health care needs, what other systems factors moderate those differences (e.g., availability of specialists, type of treatment needed, travel distance)?

## METHODS

We searched OVID MEDLINE, PsycINFO, and CINAHL, using search terms related to rural health and rural health services, for clinical trials of adult patients in the United States, published in English language, between 1990 and June, 2010. Titles and abstracts were reviewed by the authors using pre-defined exclusion criteria. Additional articles were identified by searching reference lists from relevant publications and from a search of the contents of *The Journal of Rural Health*. Study design, sample characteristic, data source, analysis, and outcome measure data were abstracted by the authors, all of whom have experience in critical analysis of the literature and who were trained on the use of the abstraction form created for this review. We created evidence tables and compiled a summary of findings for each clinical topic, and drew conclusions based on a qualitative synthesis of the findings.

## DATA SYNTHESIS

Because we wished to examine the body of evidence related to specific areas of health care, the studies were reviewed with other studies in that area. We constructed evidence tables showing the study characteristics and results for all included studies. We critically analyzed studies to compare their characteristics, methods, and findings. We compiled a summary of findings for each clinical topic, and drew conclusions based on a qualitative synthesis of the findings.

## PEER REVIEW

A draft version of this report was reviewed by nine technical experts, as well as clinical leadership. Reviewer comments were addressed and our responses were incorporated in the final report (Appendix B).

## RESULTS

We screened 1,381 unique titles and abstracts, rejected 1,048, and performed a more detailed review on 333 articles. We excluded an additional 165 articles and added 24 articles through hand-searching of references lists and *The Journal of Rural Health*. We excluded 93 articles that were not related to ambulatory care, were studies of interventions, or were useful only for background information. Three studies were added after peer-review resulting in 102 studies that reported outcomes related to one of the key questions.

The identified evidence has been presented under the following headings: preventive care/ambulatory care sensitive conditions (ACSCs), cancer care, diabetes/end stage renal disease (ESRD), cardiovascular disease, HIV/AIDS, neurologic conditions, and mental health. We also identified and presented research focused on medication use, medical procedures and tests, and provider and service utilization more generally. There are large gaps in the evidence base across clinical conditions, and minimal empirical work conducted on several areas of particular interest to the VA (e.g., traumatic brain injury, post-traumatic stress disorder, Hepatitis C).

Of the areas in which there were studies, the overall evidence base was fairly weak. In addition to a limited number of studies in most areas, only one study used a prospective design, and few linked health care differences with health outcomes. Moreover, while very large databases are needed to adequately examine many aspects of rural vs. urban health care, studies that relied on existing national or state databases were limited by the covariates available in those databases. Definitions of rural and urban vary across studies making interpretations and comparisons of findings difficult. Furthermore, many studies treated correlates of urban and rural settings as confounders and adjusted for these factors in statistical models, effectively controlling for the very factors that might underlie a potential disparity.

**Key Question #1. Do adults with health care needs who live in rural areas have different intermediate (e.g., HbA1c, Blood pressure, etc.) or final health outcomes (i.e., mortality, morbidity, QOL) than those living in urban areas?**

We identified some evidence of a health care disparity for the following conditions: suicide rates, hospitalization for ACSCs, stage of cancer presentation, and ESRD. Available evidence suggests that there is no disparity in diabetes care, the prevalence of ESRD, or control of hypertension.

**Key Question #2. Is the structure (e.g., types of available providers) or the process (e.g., likelihood of referral) of health care different for adults with health care needs who live in urban vs. rural environments?**

Urban residents tended to receive more medications but the evidence was limited. There were no consistent differences in the receipt of or adherence to medication. Office visits, medical procedures, and diagnostic tests were less frequent in rural settings, with consistently lower screening rates for breast and cervical cancer. In rural areas, cancers were more likely to be unstaged at the time of diagnosis. Rural residents were less likely to see medical specialists, including mental health specialists, and the availability of medical specialists is particularly limited in rural areas. Although rural residents were as likely as urban residents to have a usual source of care (i.e., a particular clinic), rural residents were more likely to have better continuity of care with a specific provider. Highly rural areas have an insufficient supply of health care providers, and are more likely to rely on physician extenders for primary care.

Data on quality of care were only available for a few conditions, with some evidence suggesting lower quality of care in rural areas for patients with HIV or cancer, but findings were less consistent for the treatment of depression.

**Key Question #3. If there are differences in the structure or the process of health care in rural vs. urban environments, do those differences contribute to variation in overall or intermediate health outcomes for adults with health care needs?**

Although many studies document differences in health care structure or processes, very few studies associated these differences with variation in health outcomes. Among the limited findings were higher rates of invasive cervical and breast cancers associated with lower screening rates in rural areas, improved adherence to guideline care for diabetes treatment (associated with improved access to rural health clinics), higher rates of suicide in rural areas associated with differential use of antidepressants (especially older antidepressants), and better continuity of care associated with fewer providers in rural areas.

**Key Question #4. If there are differences in intermediate or final health outcomes for adult patients with health care needs, what other systems factors moderate those differences (e.g., type of treatment needed, travel distance)?**

Other factors identified include insurance, travel distance, patient attitudes, and race disparities.

## FUTURE RESEARCH

There are many gaps in the existing research. Several important clinical conditions have not been addressed, and few studies have enrolled veterans. A key issue for future research is the choice of definitions for rural and urban areas. Researchers should provide a rationale for why a particular definition was chosen and consider using more than one definition and reporting all results. Many factors are correlated with rurality, and adjusting for all available covariates may lead to false conclusions regarding the association of rurality and study outcomes and provide insufficient information for the development of healthcare policy. For most research questions, a more contextual analytic approach should be used.

Accordingly, statistical methods should be clearly defined and researchers should report bivariate associations between rurality and study outcomes in addition to the results of multivariate models. Specific examination of rurality and race (and/or income) should be considered when appropriate, as should potential regional differences in rural-urban healthcare disparities.

Future research should move beyond documentation of differences between urban and rural health care and determine whether such differences lead to disparities in health outcomes. Studies examining health care for conditions requiring specialists or subspecialists should consider whether rural residents seek such treatment in local vs. urban settings. Across studies on rural vs. urban healthcare, prospective designs are greatly underutilized which significantly limits the strength of the evidence base.

# EVIDENCE REPORT

## INTRODUCTION

### BACKGROUND

There are approximately 3 million veterans enrolled in the VA health care system who live in rural areas (as defined by VA) -- nearly 40% of the almost 8 million veterans who are current users of VA health care.[1] Given that only 17% of the US population lives in rural areas, rural residents are disproportionately represented among veterans using VA services.[2] This trend is likely to continue, as more than one-third of OEF/OIF veterans are from rural areas.[3] The Rural Veterans Care Act of 2006 was signed into law to improve care for rural veterans. Ensuring that the health care needs of rural veterans are met has become a top priority for VA, resulting in a considerable expansion of community based outpatient clinics (CBOC's), inclusion of rural health/access as a research priority, and creation of the VA Office of Rural Health (ORH) in 2006.

A comparison of rural and urban veterans enrolled in VA health care in 1999 observed that rural veterans had lower overall health quality of life (both physical and mental), more comorbidities, and lower health quality of life within disease category than urban veterans.[4,5] Although more recent assessments have shown that rural veterans appear to have comparable or even better mental health quality of life than urban veterans, the lower physical health quality of life in rural veterans has persisted over time.[6,7] While differences in health care use between rural and urban veterans have been documented,[8] it is unclear to what extent such differences in service use contribute to the observed differences in health outcomes. Some of the rural-urban difference in physical health quality of life among VA users is likely due to differences in disease prevalence,[4] with elevated prevalence rates across numerous conditions among those rural veterans who use VA care.[9] It remains to be determined, however, whether the observed lower health quality of life among rural veterans is due to differences in disease prevalence, disparities in health care or differences in other population characteristics. Because this review focuses on health care, differences in rural-urban prevalence rates of diseases and other health conditions are beyond its scope. This systematic review examines the evidence regarding potential disparities between rural and urban areas in health care provision and delivery, and how differences in health care may contribute to disparities in health outcomes.

Our first goal was to determine if a health care disparity exists across the urban-rural spectrum. For a disparity to exist, it would have to be demonstrated that health care outcomes of patients in rural areas differ from those of patients treated in urban areas for similar conditions. Because differences in health care process or delivery do not necessarily lead to disparities, we looked for evidence associating differences with poorer health outcomes. In their report, *Unequal treatment: Confronting racial and ethnic disparities in healthcare,* the Institute of Medicine[10] defined disparity as, "…racial or ethnic differences in the quality of health care that are not due to access-related factors or clinical needs, preferences, and appropriateness of intervention"(pg 32). They go on to note, however, that inequity in care is often due to access-related factors, and that access differences are integrally tied to bias, stereotyping and inherent differences in health care systems. For the purposes of this review we conceptualized rural-urban disparities as differences in health care quality or availability.

A second goal of the review was to identify areas for intervention should any disparities be found. In order to develop a meaningful intervention, specific information regarding differences in the structure of health care and the way it is administered (i.e., the process) would be critical. Since differences in health outcomes can occur for reasons other than differences in the health care systems themselves (e.g., accessibility), our third goal was to examine what, if any, non-health care factors (e.g., travel distance to a clinic) affected health outcomes. Because veterans who use VA health care actually use more non-VA health care overall,[9] we expanded the focus of this review to include comparisons of rural vs. urban health care in non-VA health systems.

## DEFINITIONS OF RURALITY

As noted in a review of the VA rural health literature by Weeks et al. (2008),[11] synthesizing the literature on rural health is complicated by the methodologic and conceptual issues inherent in such a diverse literature. One recurrent problem is the lack of consistency across studies regarding the conventions used to define levels of rurality across communities, zip codes or counties.[11] This inconsistency affects interpretation of the individual studies as well as comparability of findings across studies.[12,13] It is beyond the scope of this review to address the complexities and ramifications of using specific population density classification schemes (for a discussion see Berke et al., 2009[14]; Stern et al., 2010[12]; West, 2010[13]). However, given the implications of this variation, we note the particular convention used to categorize rurality used in each study in the evidence tables for each section. For the convenience of readers who may be unfamiliar with these conventions, we provide a table of the most commonly used conventions along with a brief description of each (Table 1).

Table 1. Definitions of Urban and Rural (West et al. 2010;[13] Berke et al. 2009[14])

| Rural/Urban Definitions | Unit of Rural Definition | Designations | Descriptions |
|---|---|---|---|
| Office of Management and Budget (OMB) Metropolitan and Micropolitan Areas (2000) | *County Level* | | The Office of Management and Budget (OMB) Metropolitan and Micropolitan statistical areas are a county level classifications defined by the existence of an urban core, the population of the urban core, and the economic and social integration of its surrounding territory measured by commuting ties. The OMB strongly cautions against the use of Metropolitan and Micropolitan Statistical Area Standards for defining urban-rural definitions due to the fact that all counties included in Metropolitan and Micropolitan Statistical Areas and many other counties contain both urban and rural territory and populations. |
| | | Metropolitan Statistical Area | • Contains an Urbanized Area of 50,000 or more population and adjacent territory that has a high degree of social and economic integration with the core as measured by commuting ties |
| | | Micropolitan Statistical Area | • Contains an Urban Core of at least 10,000, but less than 50,000, population and adjacent territory that has a high degree of social and economic integration with the core as measured by commuting ties |
| | | Non-core based | • Based on an Urban Center of less than 10,000 people. |
| U.S. Department of Agriculture (USDA) Rural Urban Continuum Codes | *County Level* | | The 2003 USDA Rural-Urban Continuum Codes form a classification scheme that distinguishes metropolitan counties by size and nonmetropolitan counties by degree of urbanization and proximity to metro areas. This standard divides those of the Office of Management and Budget (OMB) into three metro and six non-metro categories, resulting in a 9-part county coding system. The standards for defining metropolitan areas were modified in 1958, 1971, 1975, 1980, 1990, and 2000. The current scheme was originally developed in 1974. This version allows researchers to specific populations based on population density and metro influence. Due to changes by the OMB's metro area delineation procedures for the 2000 Census, the current 2003 standards are not fully compatible with those of earlier years. |
| | | Metro | • Counties in metro areas of 1 million population or more<br>• Counties in metro areas of 250,000 to 1 million population<br>• Counties in metro areas of fewer than 250,000 population |
| | | Non-metro | • Urban population of 20,000 or more, adjacent to a metro area<br>• Urban population of 20,000 or more, not adjacent to a metro area<br>• Urban population of 2,500 to 19,999, adjacent to a metro area<br>• Urban population of 2,500 to 19,999, not adjacent to a metro area<br>• Completely rural or less than 2,500 urban population, adjacent to a metro area<br>• Completely rural or less than 2,500 urban population, not adjacent to a metro area |
| Veteran's Affairs (VA) | *County Level* | | The VA system of urban/rural classification combines those of the census blocks following census tracts urbanized areas and those of county population density. |
| | | Urban | • Urban nucleus of 50,000 or more people which may or may not contain any individual cities of 50,000 or more, but must have a core with a population density of 1,000 persons per square mile and may contain adjoining territory with at least 500 persons per square mile. |
| | | Rural | • Those counties not falling into the extremes of Urban or Highly Rural |
| | | Highly Rural | • Counties with an average population density of 7 residents per square mile |

Rural vs. Urban Ambulatory Health Care: A Systematic Review

Evidence-based Synthesis Program

| Rural/Urban Definitions | Unit of Rural Definition | Designations | Descriptions |
|---|---|---|---|
| US Dept of Agriculture Rural Urban Commuting Area codes (RUCA) | Census Tract Level | | RUCA is a 33 code system which defines rural areas in terms of census tracts based on population density in an "urban area" combined with primary and secondary commuter flow rates. Census tracts can be converted to a ZIP code approximation. Operationalization of this classification system typically involves grouping these codes into larger categories. The most common grouping uses a 4 tier system including Urban Areas, Large Rural Towns, Small Rural Towns, and Isolated Rural Towns. Below are the various versions and their data sources over time.<br>**Version 1.1** - First publicly released RUCA files. Based on 1998 ZIP code areas and 1990 Census commuting data. Data are not available.<br>**Version 1.11** - ZIP code correction made in Oregon file.<br>**Version 2.0** - Based on 2004 ZIP code areas and 2000 Census commuting data.<br><br>*An additional 2.0 version based on 2006 ZIP code areas and 2000 commuting data is also available. |
| | | Urban Areas | • ZIP codes or census tracts that have Metropolitan cores as defined by the OMB |
| | | Large Rural Towns | • ZIP codes or census tracts with Micropolitan cores and substantial commuting patterns to urban clusters |
| | | Small Rural Towns | • ZIP codes or census tracts with primary commuting flows to or within population centers of between 2,500 and 9,999 residents |
| | | Isolated Rural Towns | • ZIP codes or census tracts in less populated rural areas with no primary commuting flows to Urbanized Areas or Urban Clusters |
| U.S. Census Urban Rural Definitions | Population Density | | **2000 census criteria** All territory, population, and housing units located within an urbanized area (UA) or an urban cluster (UC). It delineates UA and UC boundaries to encompass densely settled territory, which consists of:<br>• core census block groups* or blocks that have a population density of at least 1,000 people per square mile and<br>• surrounding census blocks that have an overall density of at least 500 people per square mile<br>"Rural" therefore consists of all territory, population, and housing units located outside of UAs and UCs. Geographic entities, such as census tracts, counties, metropolitan areas, and the territory outside metropolitan areas, often are "split" between urban and rural territory, and the population and housing units they contain often are partly classified as urban and partly classified as rural.<br>**1990 census criteria** All territory, population, and housing units in urbanized areas and in places of 2,500 or more persons outside urbanized areas. More specifically, "urban" consists of territory, persons, and housing units in:<br>1. Places of 2,500 or more persons incorporated as cities, villages, boroughs (except in Alaska and New York), and towns (except in the six New England states, New York, and Wisconsin), but excluding the rural portions of "extended cities."<br>2. Census designated places of 2,500 or more persons.<br>3. Other territory, incorporated or unincorporated, included in urbanized areas. |
| | | Urbanized Area | • An urbanized area consists of a central city and surrounding areas whose population is > 50,000. They may or may not contain individual cities with 50,000 or more; rather, they must have a core with a population density generally exceeding 1,000 persons per square mile; and may contain adjoining territory with at least 500 persons per square mile (other towns outside of an urbanized area whose population exceeds 2,500). |
| | | Rural Area | • Rural areas comprise open country and settlements with fewer than 2,500 residents; areas designated as rural can have population densities as high as 999 per square mile or as low as 1 person per square mile. |
| US Dept of Agriculture Urban Influence Codes | Population Density and proximity to urban areas | | • Urban Influence Codes (2003) divide the 3,141 US counties into 12 groups combing both population density and proximity to urban areas. |
| | | Metro counties | • Divided into "large" areas with at least 1 million residents and "small" areas < 1 million residents. |
| | | Nonmetro micropolitan counties | • Divided into three groups: adjacent to a large metro area, adjacent to a small metro area, and not adjacent to a metro area. |
| | | Nonmetro noncore counties | • Divided into seven groups by: 1). their adjacency to metro or micro areas and 2) whether or not they have a town/village of at least 2,500 residents. |

*Census block group (BG) - an area normally bounded by visible features, such as streets, streams, and railroads, and by non-visible features, such as the boundary of an incorporated place.

# METHODS

## TOPIC DEVELOPMENT

This project was nominated by HSR&D and the Office of Rural Health. The analytic framework and key questions were developed with input from technical expert panel members Brian Bair, MD; John Fortney, PhD; Peter Kaboli, MD, MS; Ryan Lilly, MPA; and Alan West, PhD.

The analytic framework is depicted in Figure 1. The final key questions are:

Key Question #1. Do adults with health care needs who live in rural areas have different intermediate (e.g., HbA1c, Blood pressure, etc.) or final health care outcomes (i.e., mortality, morbidity, QOL) than those living in urban areas?

Key Question #2. Is the structure (e.g., types of available providers) or the process (e.g., likelihood of referral) of health care different for adults with health care needs who live in urban vs. rural environments?

Key Question #3. If there are differences in the structure or the process of health care in rural vs. urban environments, do those differences contribute to variation in overall or intermediate health outcomes for adults with health care needs?

Key Question #4. If there are differences in intermediate or final health outcomes for adult patients with health care needs, what systems factors other than those due to differences in health care structure or process moderate those differences (e.g., travel distance)?

## SEARCH STRATEGY

We searched OVID MEDLINE, PsycINFO, and CINAHL from 1990 to June, 2010 using the following MEDLINE search terms (or the corresponding terms in PsycINFO and CINAHL): hospitals, rural; rural health; rural population; rural health services, and United States. Limits to the search included English language, published 1990 or later, population age of 18 years or older, and publication types randomized controlled trial, clinical trial, cohort or cross-sectional study, meta-analysis, or review. Additionally, we did a hand search of references lists of relevant articles and of *The Journal of Rural Health* using the limits noted above.

**Figure 1. Analytic Framework**

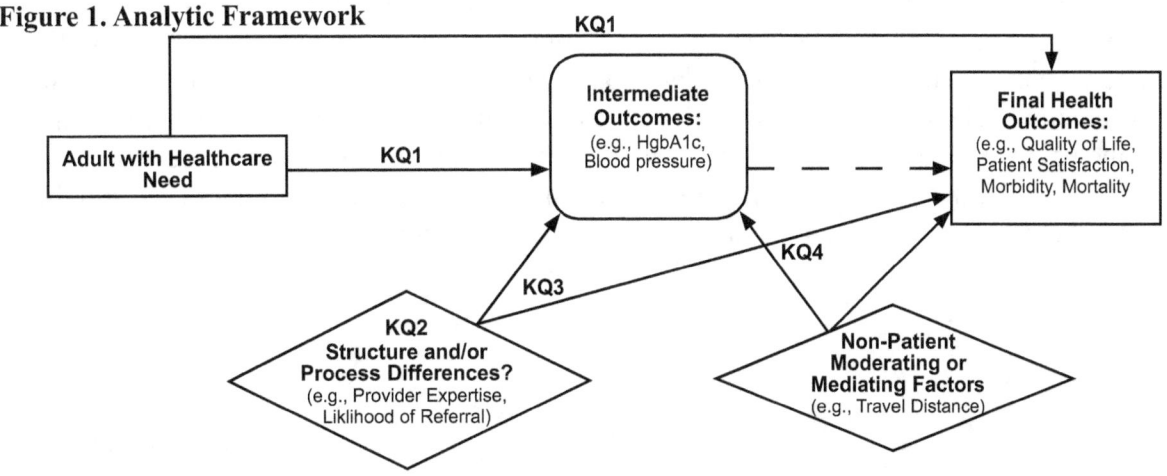

## STUDY SELECTION

The principal investigator, co-investigators, and one of the research associates, all with experience in critical review of published studies, reviewed abstracts of articles identified in the search and selected articles for further review based on pre-defined exclusion criteria. In addition to the exclusion criteria used to limit the search, we also excluded articles if they were not about health care (e.g., focused on disease prevalence), if they did not include patients from rural settings, or if they were not about ambulatory care. Eligible articles provided primary data relevant to the key questions.

## DATA ABSTRACTION

Data from eligible articles was abstracted by the principal investigator, co-investigators, and one of the research associates onto a brief screening form (see Appendix A). The principal investigator developed the form and all abstractors completed forms for a common set of six articles. Results of the trial abstraction were reviewed with the principal investigator. The abstraction form captured data on the study design, sample (including whether the subjects in the study were Veterans), definition of rural used in the study, data source including the date of datesets used, analyses including covariates, and outcome measures.

## DATA SYNTHESIS

Because we wished to examine the body of evidence related to specific areas of health care, the studies were reviewed with other studies in that area. We constructed evidence tables showing the study characteristics and results for all included studies. We critically analyzed studies to compare their characteristics, methods, and findings. We compiled a summary of findings for each clinical topic, and drew conclusions based on a qualitative synthesis of the findings.

## RATING THE BODY OF EVIDENCE

Due to the qualitative nature of the synthesis, standard methods for rating the body of evidence do not apply and there are no validated rating systems to compare the quality of observational studies. Based on the work of others,[15,16,17] we developed a rating system that we used as a heuristic in our efforts to compare studies that used different methodologies and to facilitate a synthesis of the evidence base in each content area. Although these ratings are essentially qualitative in nature, they provide the reader with information regarding our evaluations of the studies and, consequently, the overall evidence base. For each study, we evaluated the internal and the external validity, and then assigned an overall Confidence Score based on these ratings. The principal investigator and one of the co-investigators rated all articles after independently rating a set of 20 articles and reviewing the results. In Table 2 we detail the scales used and the kinds of elements that were considered within each rating category.

**Table 2. Explanation of Confidence Scores**

| Internal Validity | Rated G(Good), F(Fair), P(Poor). In order to receive a "G" for internal validity would need to have "G" ratings for all subsumed elements. |
|---|---|
| Sampling Method/Bias | Low response rates without correction; convenience sampling; |
| Predictors/Confounders | Omission of socioeconomic/insurance factors or other factors usually associated with service use (e.g., age). |
| Outcomes | Unreliable or not validated measures; use of proxy variables (e.g., self-reported service use) |
| Statistical Methods | Omission of bivariate or multivariate statistics; Ignored data clustering |
| **External Validity** | Rated G(Good), F(Fair), P(Poor). In order to receive a "G" for external validity would need to have "G" ratings for all subsumed elements. |
| Use of proxy variables or aggregate measures | Use of county level predictors or outcomes in lieu of individual ones; Dichotomized urban rural without further gradations if urban/rural were a covariate in their model. |
| Representativeness of sample | Small samples; samples limited to one demographic group; no correction for biased sampling; |
| Study design appropriate for the research question? | Dichotomized urban rural without further gradations if area of residence was the focus of the study; poorly conceptualized study; data insufficient to answer primary research question. |
| **Overall Confidence Score** | Rated as follows:<br>*High Quality* = further research unlikely to change confidence in effects. *Both internal and external rated as "G"*<br>*Moderate Quality*= further research likely to have an important impact on confidence and may change the estimate of effect.<br>*Low Quality*= further research is very likely to have an important impact and will likely change the estimate of effect.<br>*Very Low Quality*= any estimate of effect is uncertain.<br><br>Note: "H" Overall Confidence Score would require "Good" ratings for both Internal and External Validity. |

# PEER REVIEW

A draft version of this report was sent to nine peer reviewers. Their comments and our responses are presented in Appendix B.

# RESULTS

## LITERATURE FLOW

The literature flow is presented in Figure 2. The combined search library contained 1,381 citations, of which we reviewed 333 articles at the full-text level. We excluded 165 of the 333 articles and added 24 references through hand-searching reference lists of relevant articles and *The Journal of Rural Health*. Of 192 possible studies, we excluded 93 because they were not related to ambulatory care, described an intervention, or provided background information. Three studies were added based on comments received during peer-review resulting in 102 articles reporting data pertaining to one of the key questions. The included articles were categorized under the following ambulatory care services: preventive care/ambulatory care sensitive conditions, cancer care, diabetes/end stage renal disease, cardiovascular disease, HIV/AIDS, neurologic conditions, and mental health. We also identified and included articles focused on use of medication, medical procedures and tests, and provider and service utilization more generally.

**Figure 2. Flow Diagram of Included Studies**

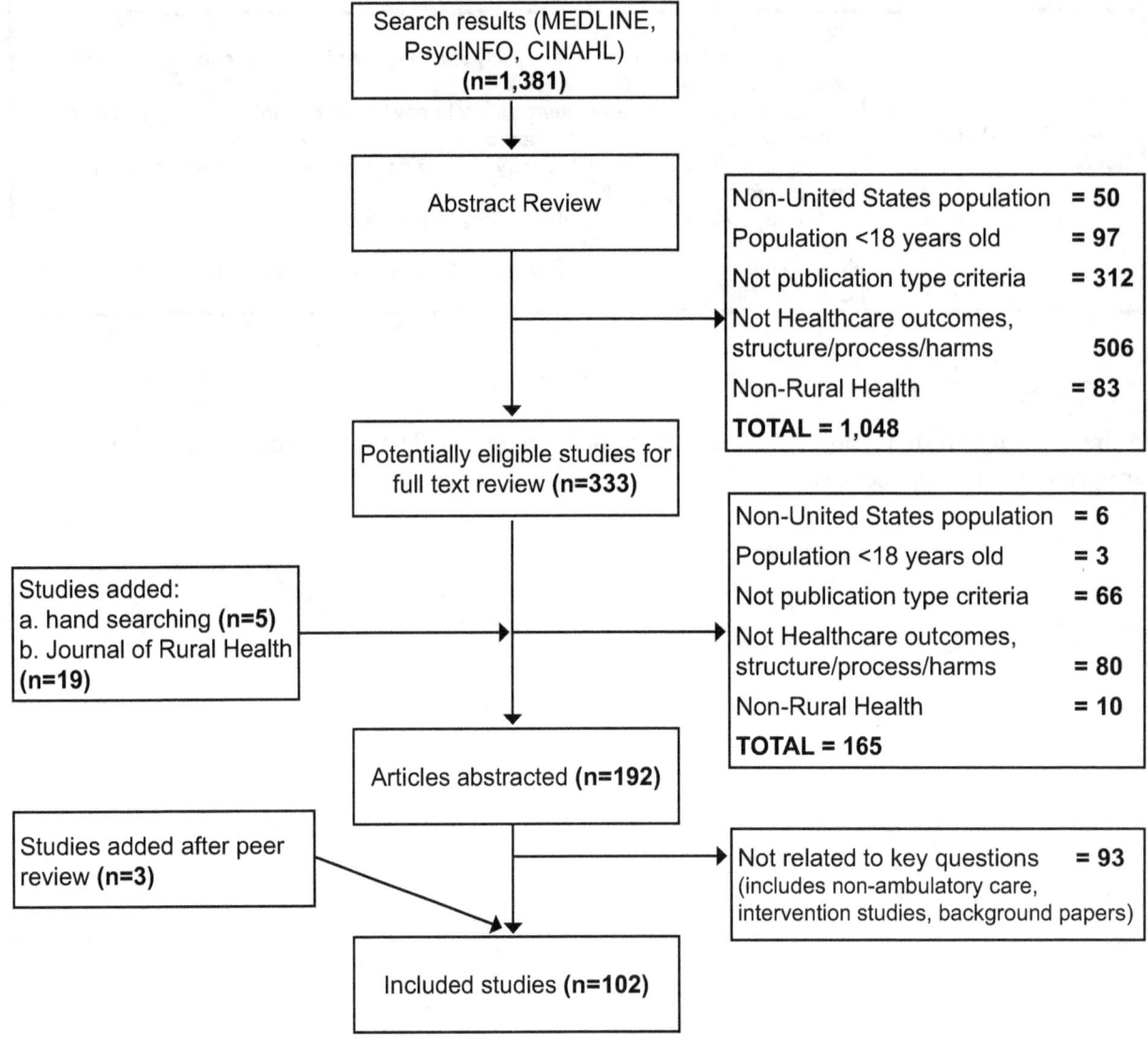

## PREVENTIVE CARE/AMBULATORY CARE SENSITIVE CONDITIONS (Table 3 and Appendix C, Tables 1 and 2)

There were two studies looking at immunization rates,[18,19] nine looking at cancer screening rates,[18-26] one examining prenatal care,[27] and three examining hospital rates for ambulatory care sensitive conditions.[28-30]

Immunization rates were examined in only two studies, both using data more than 10 years old. Among respondents to the 1994 US National Health Interview Survey, the rate of flu shot receipt among 4,051 people over 65 yr was examined.[19] No differences were observed between older rural and urban residents in the receipt of flu vaccine in adjusted analyses. Similarly, national data of 130,452 respondents from the 1997 Behavioral Risk Factor Surveillance System (BRFSS) and the 1999 Area Resource File found no rural-urban differences in the rates of either flu or pneumonia vaccines among women age 65 years and older.[18]

Only one study examined prenatal care.[27] This study used the 2003 Oregon Pregnancy Risk Assessment Monitoring System to examine the odds of receiving prenatal care after the first trimester in RUCA defined urban, large rural and small rural areas among 1,508 women. Women were surveyed post childbirth about when during their pregnancy they initiated prenatal care (if at all). No differences were found between residence categories in the odds of late initiation (after first trimester) of prenatal care. However, given methodologic problems with the study, our confidence in this finding is moderately low.

Ambulatory care sensitive conditions (ACSC) are those conditions in which inadequate outpatient treatment leads to increases in hospitalization.[30] Conditions that are considered to be ambulatory care sensitive include congestive heart failure (CHF), hypertension, angina, chronic obstructive pulmonary disease, as well as other conditions in which hospitalization can usually be avoided, such as bacterial pneumonia, cellulitis, diabetes, gastroenteritis, asthma, and urinary tract infections. A study of the prevalence of ACSC hospital admissions in New York State from 1991-1993 found that the rates increased as population density decreased within each of the demographic groupings (New York City area, upstate urban-suburban areas, more remote rural). They did not compare across areas. Of note, the percentage of blacks was positively associated with the rate of ACSC admissions in the two more populous groupings.[30] In a much better designed study, Laditka (2009) examined ACSC admissions in 8 states during 2002.[28] They reported a step-wise increase in the rate ratios of admissions for patients 18-64 years across levels of rurality adjusted for demographics and availability of health care services. Although further adjustment for death rates from chronic diseases (e.g., heart disease) did not change the association appreciably, adjustment for percentage of population that was uninsured reduced the association across all levels of population density, suggesting that insurance-related access contributed to the variation across the spectrum of population density. However, since rates in the most rural areas remain elevated relative to urban rates even after adjusting for insurance (RR=1.28, 95%CI=1.12-1.47) the contribution of insurance possession to the population density effect is only partial. For patients 65 years or older, the step-wise increase in ACSC admissions was retained when all adjustments were made except for those related to death rates and physician supply (which was not significantly associated with ACSC admissions) (RR=1.46, 95%CI=1.39-1.52 most rural:urban).

A study of secondary and tertiary prevention among 787 older adults with ACSCs (specifically, arthritis, hypertension, coronary heart disease, diabetes mellitus, peptic ulcer disease, and chronic obstructive pulmonary disease [COPD]), was conducted in Iowa in 1995.[29] No differences were found between rural and urban residents in condition-specific prevention scores, but methodologic limitations of this study resulted in a low Confidence Score, suggesting that these results are likely to change with new information. Although rural residents with these chronic conditions saw fewer specialists than urban residents (7% vs. 12%, p<0.05), and were somewhat less likely to report a need for medical advice in the previous year (50% vs. 58%, p<0.05), they also had better continuity of care than urban residents (100% vs. 83% of time seeing physician they saw most, p<0.001).

The rate of colorectal cancer (CRC) screening was assessed in two national studies, and one regional study. All three studies found a rural disadvantage in screening rates. National data of 130,452 respondents from the 1997 Behavioral Risk Factor Surveillance System (BRFSS) and the 1999 Area Resource File examined CRC screens (fecal occult blood test or proctosigmoidoscopy). Residents from rural areas adjacent or non-adjacent to urban areas were less likely to get CRC screening (ORs=0.83 and 0.82, respectively).[18] Similar results were reported using the 1998-1999 datasets of the BRFSS of 23,565 men and 37,847 women over age 50 years.[22] In rural areas, 16.2% of residents had a fecal occult blood test vs. 22% in large urban areas. Examining sigmoidoscopy/colonoscopy rates yielded a similar finding, with 28.2% of rural residents receiving these screens vs. 35.2% of those who live in large urban areas. Although attenuated, these differences remained after adjustments. A case-control study of CRC screening in North Carolina using a nurse led patient interview found fewer rural residents reported CRC screening in the previous 5 years.[24] When differences in screening rates were held constant, a rural disparity in the incidence of CRC was eliminated, suggesting a difference in health care access.

There were five studies examining breast and cervical cancer screening rates in national samples. The 1994 US National Health Interview Survey was used to assess, cervical and breast cancer screening (i.e., mammography) among 8,970 age 18 years and older, and among 2,729 women age 50 years and older respectively.[19] No differences were observed between rural and urban women in the receipt of cervical cancer screens. Differences were found between urban and rural women in mammography (68% of urban vs. 61 percent of rural; p =0.01). These differences were no longer apparent after adjustment for education, household income and health insurance status. Among the 12,637 patients 65 yr and older and/or disabled who participated in the 1993 Medicare Current Beneficiary Survey, screening rates were lower among women from smaller non-urban counties relative to large urban counties for breast (28.6% vs. 34.4%) and cervical (28.4% vs. 23.1%) cancers in bivariate analyses.[26] As with the 1994 National Health Interview study, these differences disappeared after adjusting for income, Medicaid status, physician availability, age, race, education and functional status.

All three studies using the BRFSS datasets found rural-urban differences in breast and/or cervical screening rates. In a study using the 1997 BRFSS database,[18] women from rural areas were significantly less likely to get cervical cancer screening (ORs=0.86 and 0.88), while only those from rural areas adjacent to metropolitan areas were less likely to get mammograms (OR=0.82). Factors found to be predictive of screenings included insurance status, availability of primary care providers, and income. A study using the 1998-1999 BRFSS database examined mammography and clinical breast exams among 108,326 women over 40 years old, and cervical cancer screens among 131,813 women over the age of 18 years.[21] Among rural women over 40 years old, 66.7% had mammograms and 73% had clinical breast exams. The rates among urban women were 75.4% for mammography and 78.2% for clinical breast exams. Similar differences for cervical cancer screening rates were found, with 81.3% of rural women and 84.5% of the most urban women getting screens. These differences were attenuated with adjustment, but remained significant. Of note, rural-urban differences were greater among black and Hispanic women. Finally, a study examining cervical screening rates using 2002 BRFSS, found that the odds of receiving a Pap test among 91,492 rural women depended on the number of available primary care providers.[23] Urban women who lived in counties with fewer providers (i.e., fewer than 300 primary providers per 100,000 women) were more likely to get a Pap test than rural or suburban women from counties with similar provider availability (OR=1.13, 95%CI=1-1.28). In counties in which there were moderate numbers of providers (i.e., 300-500 per 100,000 women), only those in suburban counties were disadvantaged (OR=0.72, 95%CI=0.55-0.94). The odds of mammogram receipt were greater for urban (OR=1.21, 95%CI=1.11-1.32) and suburban (OR=1.28, 95%CI=1.17-1.4) women than rural women independent of provider availability.

In both regional studies in which breast and cervical cancer screening rates were assessed there was a rural disadvantage, though significance remained after adjustment in only one of the studies. Using state BRFSS data from 1996-1997, non-disabled rural women in Iowa were found to have had lower rates of screening for breast ($X^2$=5.73, p<0.0001) and cervical ($X^2$=6.0, p<0.0001) cancer than their urban counterparts.[25] For example, of those from the most rural regions (population density of fewer than 20 people per square mile), only 37.3% received a mammogram and only 61.3% were screened for cervical cancer. In contrast, in the most densely populated areas (100 or more per square mile), 56.4% and 73.7% received screenings for breast and cervical cancers respectively. Similarly, a smaller study using 1,922 respondents from the Tennessee BRFSS for 2001 and 2003 found more urban than rural women received a mammogram in the previous two years (78.3%, 95%CI=75.9-80.7 vs. 71.3%, 95%CI=67.4-75.2).[20] After adjusting for demographics, insurance status and having a health care provider, however, rural residence status was no longer significant.

## Summary

Immunization rates appear to be comparable in rural vs. urban areas; however, given that there were only two studies and that both relied on data 10 years old, our confidence in this finding while moderate, remains provisional.

The one study of prenatal care suggested no rural-urban difference; however, given the study design, the regional nature of the sample and the absence of confirmatory findings, our confidence in the evidence base is low.

All studies examining cancer screening rates found rural-urban differences. The primary difference among the studies was that in some of them, the rural-urban difference disappeared once access factors (e.g., income, availability of physicians, insurance status) were controlled, while in others the differences remained significant albeit of a smaller magnitude. This suggests that rural-urban differences in cancer screening rates are at least partially due to differences in health care access.

Of note, screening rates are not uniformly lower across rural areas. For example, a study looking at rates of mammography in randomly selected Rural Health Clinics nationally found triple the rate of screening in the Middle third of the country compared to that in the Western third of the country (OR=3.75, 95%CI=1.43-9.87).[31] Studies using national databases, therefore, may overlook actual rural-urban differences by pooling across regions.

Hospitalizations associated with ACSCs are, at best, indirect measures of health care quality and/or access. Of the two studies examining hospitalization rates for ACSCs, we had greater confidence in the study that sampled from eight states and in which a higher rate of hospitalization for these conditions was found in rural areas. That the presence of federally qualified Rural Health Clinics or Community Health Centers have been found in other studies to diminish the rates of ACSC hospital admissions,[32] suggests that such admissions may be related to the availability of health care resources. Still, given the limited evidence base, this can only be viewed as provisional.

**Table 3. Confidence Scores for Preventive Care/Ambulatory Care Sensitive Condition Studies**

| Study | Casey 2001[18] | Zhang 2000[19] | Kinney 2006[24] | Epstein 2009[27] | Laditka 2009[28] | Schreiber 1997[30] | Saag 1998[29] 18 | Coughlin 2002[21] | Coughlin 2004[22] | Coughlin 2008[23] | Stearns 2000[26] | Brown 2009[20] | Schootman 1999[25] |
|---|---|---|---|---|---|---|---|---|---|---|---|---|---|
| **Internal Validity** | G | G | G | F | G | F | F | G | G | G | G | G | G |
| Sampling Method/Bias | G | G | G | F | G | G | F | G | G | G | G | G | G |
| Predictors/Confounders | G | G | G | G | G | F | G | G | G | G | G | G | G |
| Outcomes | G | G | G | F/P | G | G | F | G | G | G | G | G | G |
| Statistical Methods | G | G | G | G | G | F | G | G | G | G | G | G | G |
| **External Validity** | G | F | G | F | F | F | F | G | G | G | F | F | F |
| Use of proxy variables or aggregate measures | G | G | G | G | F | F | F | G | G | G | G | G | F |
| Sample Representativeness (size, composition) | G | F | G | F | G | G | G | G | G | G | F | G | G |
| Design appropriate for the research question | G | G | F | G | G | F | G | G | G | G | G | F | F |
| **Overall Confidence Score** | H | M | M | M/L | M | L | L | H | H | H | M | M | M |

## CANCER CARE (Table 4 and Appendix C, Table 3)

Comparisons of rural and urban health care for cancer have focused on variation in staging, mortality, and quality of care. There were 12 studies comparing urban and rural cancer care. Three studies examined mortality.[25,33,34] Nine studies examined cancer stage at the time of diagnosis,[24,25,33,35-40] three studies examined the relationship between screening and disease progression,[25,35,37] and five looked at treatment quality.[33-35,41,42]

Of the three studies of mortality, two were of regional samples and the one national study used a sample of people 65 years and older. Using the Iowa Surveillance, Epidemiology, and End

Results (SEER) database for 1991-1995 and the BFRSS database for 1996-1997, mortality among breast and cervical cancer patients was examined.[25] No differences in age adjusted mortality rates for cervical and breast cancer were found between rural and urban women. Similarly, using the national SEER database and the Medicare Claims database from 1995 and 1999, patients over 65 years with lung cancer were identified and service utilization, stage of illness at presentation and mortality rates were compared across four levels of rurality (N=26,073).[33] As in the Iowa study, no differences were seen in overall survival between rural and urban areas either before or after adjustments. Factors that were predictive of mortality were patient demographics, receipt of radiation for those with stage II and IV disease, and the number of subspecialists per 10,000 residents 65 years and older. Both the odds of radiation receipt and the supply of subspecialists were lower in rural areas (radiation 47.0% urban vs. 43.2% rural, trend only; subspecialists: urban 10.6 ±7.6 per 10,000 residents vs. most rural 1.2 ± 3.3 per 10,000, p<0.01).

Mortality was also evaluated in a cohort of patients with lymphoma diagnoses who were registered in the Nebraska Medical Center Oncology Database.[34] Overall survival rates were lower for those rural residents who were treated by community providers as compared to either urban residents or rural residents treated by university affiliated providers (5 year survival rate 51% vs. 59-66%; p<0.001), suggesting that community providers in rural areas had less expertise. However, because of the nature of the sample used, this finding may not be generalizeable.

Four studies examined differences in rates of diagnostic staging at the time of initial cancer presentation.[33,35,37,38] Three studies found differences between rural and urban areas in the odds of having an incident cancer staged, whereas one national study of lung cancer patients 65 years and older did not find differential odds between rural and urban areas.[33] A comparison of 1,105 urban residents and 1,463 rural residents from 18 rural communities surrounding Lake Superior with incident cancer between 1992-1997,[35] found that rural cancer patients were less likely to have breast (60% vs. 83%), prostate (41% v. 60%) or non-small cell lung cancers (82% vs. 90%) staged at the time of initial diagnosis than urban residents. No differences were found in rate of staging for prostate or small cell lung cancers. Examination of 9,685 new cancer cases recorded in the Mississippi State Department of Health Central Cancer Registry in 1996 found that rural residents had significantly lower odds of having their lung, colorectal, breast or prostate cancers staged at the time of diagnosis (OR=0.83)[37]. This rural disadvantage was notably more pronounced for women (OR=0.75) and for African Americans (OR=0.73). Controlling for race and gender, rural white males were less likely to have their prostate cancer staged than were urban white males (OR=0.70). Finally, a national study of lung and colorectal cancer (CRC) patients found decreased odds of cancer staging at the time of diagnosis among rural residents.[38] In a study of 129,811 colorectal cancer patients and 161,479 lung cancer patients registered in the SEER database between 2000-2003, rural patients were less likely to have had their cancer staged for both lung (14% vs. 9%) and colorectal (9% vs. 6%) cancers.[38] Taken together, the data suggest differences between rural and urban residents in the odds of having unstaged disease. Moreover, the lower rate of incident cancer staging at the time of presentation may vary by race, geographic location, type of cancer and age of the patient.

Studies that examined stage of disease progression at the time of diagnosis used this outcome so as to infer differences in screening rates and/or treatment access not captured in most national and state databases. For example, examination of the rate of *in situ* vs. invasive breast and cervical cancers recorded in the Iowa SEER database between 1991-1995 showed that women who were from more urban areas had higher age-adjusted rates of *in situ* breast cancer (47.7 vs. 37.3 per 100,000) and lower rates of invasive cervical cancer (7.3 vs. 9.3 per 100,000), both of which were interpreted as indicating underutilization of screening in rural areas.[25] Similarly, among 2,568 cancer patients in the Lake Superior area study who were staged at the time of diagnosis, rural residents with breast, colorectal, and non-small cell lung cancers were more likely to present at later stages of disease progression than urban residents with those conditions.[35] Staging differences were not noted for prostate or small cell lung cancers, however. The Mississippi study also found that rural residents were more likely to present with regional or distant metastatic disease (vs. local) compared to urban residents when cancer types were considered collectively ($X^2$=8.4, df=2, p<0.05).[37] Comparisons within cancer types in the Mississippi study found that differences between rural and urban residents in the risk for more advanced disease was significant only for lung cancer ($X^2$=12.3, p<0.005).[37]

In contrast to these findings, several studies reported no rural-urban differences or reported an urban disadvantage, and only one of them received a low confidence score.[36] For example, the national study of Medicare beneficiaries 65 years and older by Shugarman (2008),[33] found no differences between urban and rural areas in the stage of lung cancer at the time of diagnosis, nor did a case-control study of CRC in North Carolina.[24] A large national study of colorectal (n=129,811) and lung (n=161,479) cancers using the SEER database compared the odds of late stage disease presentation between the RUCC-defined highly urban and most rural areas (population less than 20,000).[38] Relative to the rural areas, *urban* residence was associated with a small but significantly increased likelihood of stage IV disease for both colorectal (17.9% rural vs. 18.5% urban) and lung (41.2% rural vs. 42.9% urban) cancers after controlling for race, age, median county income and gender. A large study using a multi-level modeling approach to examine the odds of late stage initial presentations of breast, colorectal, lung, and prostate cancers among over 140,000 patients in the Illinois State Cancer Registry who developed cancer between 1998-2002 also found that urban residents were more likely to present with later stage disease for all four cancer types.[39]

In the Illinois study,[39] disparities between urban and rural areas for prostate cancer were eliminated when the model included the patient factors of race and age. For colorectal cancer, the urban disadvantage partially disappeared in the model including patient age and race (B= -0.156, p<0.05 for the most rural) and almost completely disappeared in the model including income and access (B= -0.085, p>0.05 for the most rural). This suggests that distance from a healthcare provider, being young and black were risk factors for later stage of presentation for this illness. Only residence in large towns was associated with lower odds for later stage disease presentation (B= -0.198, p<0.05). For breast cancer, those who were in the most rural areas were equally likely as those in metropolitan Chicago to present with late stage disease (B= - 0.032, p >0.05) and, similar to colorectal cancer, the greatest advantage was for residents of large towns (B= -0.167, p<0.05). Rural areas were comparable to urban areas once age and race were included in the model. Only lung cancer showed a clear urban disadvantage in each model, the greatest advantage being for those residents who were diagnosed in large towns (B= -0.431, p<0.05), a finding similar to that for breast and colorectal cancers.

The advantage for large rural towns in the Illinois study was also found in a well designed study of cancer patients in Nebraska. Examination of the stage of cancer at the time of diagnosis among 5,521 incident colorectal cancers in Nebraska between 1998-2003 found that residents from micropolitan communities (i.e., counties with an urban cluster of 10,000 to 49,999 people) were more likely to present with CRC at earlier stages of disease than residents from more rural or more urban areas in both adjusted and unadjusted analyses (OR=1.22, 95%CI=1.05, 1.42).[40]

There were very few studies examining the quality of cancer care and those that did suggest that there may be lower quality care in rural areas. Elliott (2004) reported that rural treatment of cancer was found to be of lower quality in the Great Lakes region across cancer types in terms of initial management, clinical trial participation and post-treatment surveillance; however, scores derived to measure these variables were not independently validated.[35] In a study of almost 7,000 women treated for breast cancer from 1991-1996 in the national SEER database, younger women with newly diagnosed ductal carcinoma *in situ* had reduced odds of therapeutic radiation receipt if they lived in a rural area (OR=0.38).[42] While radiation receipt among younger women was not related to availability of therapeutic radiation in the patient's county, for older women more distant access to a therapeutic radiation site was associated with reduced odds of radiation receipt (OR=0.48). A similar finding was observed in a national study of Medicare beneficiaries over 65 years, where fewer of those living in rural areas received radiation (most urban 46.8% vs most rural 43.2%).[33]

Two studies observed differences in the availability of cutting edge treatments, but since both studies were rated with fairly low Confidence Scores the findings should only be viewed as suggestive and worthy of further study. A study of 461 women with estrogen sensitive breast cancers listed in the North Carolina Central Cancer Registry and who were also Medicaid enrollees between 2000-2004 examined the odds of ever receiving a prescription for an aromatase inhibitor (vs. Tamoxifen only). Rural residents were less likely than urban patients to have received a prescription for an aromatase inhibitor (OR=0.54).[41] The quality of lymphoma treatment was found to be lagging in rural areas, but only if the provider was not university affiliated.[34] While this suggests that rural community based treatment for lymphoma is of lower quality, our confidence in the generalizability of these findings is relatively low.

## Summary

The evidence for differences in cancer-related health outcomes related to place of residence is relatively weak for most outcomes. Many of the studies used data that were at least 10 years old. Given the rapidly evolving nature of oncologic care, this is a significant limitation.

There were no consistent rural-urban differences in mortality or in the stage of illness at the time of initial presentation. Greater consistency was noted in the odds of unstaged disease, with rural residents less likely to have their cancer staged at the time of initial presentation. Interpretation of this finding is complicated by two factors, however. First, studies categorized patients by residence rather than by point of care and rural patients are more likely to pursue treatment for conditions such as cancer in urban areas.[43] Rural providers may not pursue diagnostic procedures necessary to stage cancer if the patient intends to pursue treatment elsewhere. Second, the evidence base may be subject to a reporting bias since the odds of cancer staging were never the primary focus of the studies reviewed and studies that did not find a difference may not have reported a null finding.

It must be noted that patients in rural areas are not homogeneous, and barriers impeding screening of and treatment for cancer vary within both urban and rural populations. Depending on the compositions of the rural and urban samples being compared, age differences, income factors and racial/ethnic disparities may underlie some rural-urban differences when they emerge. For example, the large percentage of low income blacks in Chicago relative to the more rural areas in Illinois likely contributed to urban disadvantage in the odds of later stage of cancer at initial presentation. Similarly, older breast cancer patients may be more affected by distance to care than younger patients.

Finally, studies looking at rural-urban differences in quality of care were few and methodologically problematic given either a lack of association with specific treatment guidelines or that treatment guidelines changed during the course of the study (e.g., McLaughlin, 2009).[41]

**Table 4. Confidence Scores for Cancer Care Studies**

| Study | Shugarman 2008[33] | Loberiza 2009[34] | Elliott 2004[35] | Paquette 2007[38] | Higginbotham 2001[37] | Chirumbole 2009[36] | Schootman 1999[25] | Kinney 2006[24] | Sankaranarayanan 2009[40] | McLafferty 2009[39] | Schootman 2001[42] | McLaughlin 2009[41] |
|---|---|---|---|---|---|---|---|---|---|---|---|---|
| **Internal Validity** | G | F | F | F | F | F | G | G | G | G/F | F | F |
| Sampling Method/Bias | G | F | G | G | G | G | G | G | G | G | G | G |
| Predictors/Confounders | G | F | G | F | F | F | G | G | G | G/F | F | G |
| Outcomes (clarity of measurement) | G | G | F | G | G | F | G | G | G | G | G | F |
| Statistical Methods | G | G | G | G | F | F | G | G | G | G | G | G |
| **External Validity** | F | F | F | F | F | F | F | G | G/F | F | F | F |
| Use of proxy variables or aggregate measures | G | G | G/F | G | G | F | G | G | G | F | F | G |
| Representativeness of sample | F | F/P | G | F | G | G | G | G | G | G | G | F/P |
| Study design appropriate for the research question? | G | G | F | G | F | F | F | F | G/F | G | G | G |
| **Overall Confidence Score** | M | M/L | M/L | M | M | L | M | M | H/M | M | M | M/L |

## DIABETES/END STAGE RENAL DISEASE (Table 5 and Appendix C, Table 4)

Only three studies (all cross-sectional) examined potential differences in health outcomes between urban and rural residents for diabetes or kidney disease.[44-46] One moderate to high quality study relied on patient self-report to assess complications of diabetes in a national sample,[45] while a low quality examined the incidence of diabetes-related end-stage renal disease.[46] The third study, of high quality, examined mortality rates between urban and rural patients receiving dialysis.[44] There were six studies (also all cross-sectional) examining differences in measures of care for diabetes (e.g., concordance with American Diabetes Association [ADA] guidelines). Two were of low quality, two were of moderate quality, and two were of moderate to high quality. The smallest study compared two sites,[47] two national studies reported no difference between rural and urban areas,[48,49] and another large national study reported a mixed effect of residence category in that some outcome measures were more favorable for those in rural areas whereas others were more favorable for those in urban areas.[45] A fifth study in Washington State found better quality of care measures in large towns than in either urban or more rural areas.[50] The sixth study of adherence to ADA guideline recommendations was a national study that found rural disparities, but only in some parts of the country, and rural advantage in others.[51]

In a study by Morden et al. (2010),[49] quality indicators of eye exams, foot exams, LDL levels, blood pressure and hemoglobin A1c (HbA1c) levels were assessed among 11,688 veterans with diabetes in 2005. No differences were found in quality indicators between highly rural and urban RUCA categories. Koopman (2006), using the National Health and Nutrition Examination Survey from 1988-1994 and rural or urban classification based on metropolitan statistical areas, found that urban Hispanics had higher odds of their diabetes not being detected relative to urban whites (3.7% vs. 2.3%), rural whites (2.8%), and rural Hispanics (2.7%; $p<0.05$).[45] Urban Hispanics were also more likely than the other groups to report a lack of usual source of health care (11.4% vs. 1.8% urban whites, 6.5% rural whites, and 5.1% rural Hispanics; $p<0.01$). In multivariate analyses, urban vs. rural primary residence was not associated with the odds of diabetes being detected once demographic and health care utilization were controlled. This further supports the association between non-detection of diabetes and limited contact with health care providers. In addition, rural Hispanics more frequently had uncontrolled BP relative to urban Hispanics (OR=1.5, 95%CI=0.94-3.45) or either group of whites ($p<0.01$), but they were not significantly different from either group of whites in multivariate analyses controlling for demographic, access and some health factors. There were no group differences in glycemic or control or lipid levels.

A rural disadvantage was reported in a very small study in Alabama comparing patients in one "rural" family practice clinic (n=78) and one "urban" internal medicine clinic (n=109) with respect to HbA1c levels, eye exams, foot exams, lipid profiles, and microalbuminuria tests.[47] Urban and rural were not defined, and given the local nature of the study and the methodologic issues, our confidence in this finding is very low.

A much larger and better designed study comparing compliance with ADA guidelines for HbA1c levels, eye exams, and foot exams in two national databases reported that rural residents with diabetes received both more and less guideline care depending on the outcome and database used.[45] Although the directions of effects were the same in both databases, they were only significantly different in the larger database. Slightly more rural residents, defined as those living in non-metropolitan statistical areas, received a quarterly HbA1c level (OR=1.16), but this difference was no longer significant after adjustments (i.e., race, region of the country, insurance coverage, and having a personal physician). Differences that remained significant even after adjustment were decreased odds among rural diabetics of having a dilated eye exam (OR=0.88) or foot exam (OR=0.85) or receiving diabetes education (OR=0.83). Inconsistent evidence for rural-urban differences in diabetes care was reported in a study of older Medicare patients in Washington State.[50] Urban residents with diabetes were equally as likely as rural residents to get eye exams, but they were more likely than rural residents (defined based on RUCA with 4 rural subgroups) to get an HbA1c check (55.6% vs. 52.2%) and a cholesterol screen (66.6% vs. 63.2%). After adjustments, residents living in large remote rural towns were the most likely to have had the tests. Importantly, rural residents were only less likely to get the assessments if they had not seen an endocrinologist in the prior year.[50] That is, specialty consultation, much more common among urban residents, was a primary determinant as to whether patients received the guideline assessments.

Some of the inconsistency across studies may be due to differences between rural and urban areas in the rate of adherence to guideline recommended tests across geographic regions of the country. For example, in an examination of the geographic distribution of diabetic patients receiving a composite measure of guideline tests (i.e., lipid levels, HbA1c levels, and eye exams), Weingarten et al. (2006), found that rural residents (categorized as rural or semi-rural) were actually more likely to receive the tests than urban residents depending on in which region of the country they lived.[51] Because the study relied on aggregate measures, however, this finding should be considered only tentative.

One of the many deleterious consequences of poorly controlled diabetes is end-stage renal disease (ESRD). Ward (2009) compared the rural and urban zip codes of 18,377 diabetic patients in California for the odds of ESRD attributable to diabetes.[46] There was only a trend for a decreased likelihood of ESRD among rural patients (beta=-0.035, p<0.06). However, because the model was adjusted for factors associated with access and poor illness control (i.e., insurance status and number of hospitalizations due to hyperglycemic complications), it may be that one of these factors underlies the differences associated with rural vs. urban residence. That patients from health professional shortage areas were actually less likely to have ESRD, may reflect this problem with their model. Because bivariate results were not reported for this parameter, we could not assess potential problems with the statistical model used and rated our confidence in the finding as low.

In an analysis of treatment for 552,279 patients with ESRD who initiated dialysis between 1995-2002, the impact of rural vs. urban residence varied by race and ethnicity.[44] There were no significant differences between urban and rural areas in types of treatment other than that rural areas (including large rural, small rural, and remote) were more likely to use peritoneal dialysis. When target hematocrit levels were the outcome, there were no significant differences between urban and rural areas. Target urea reduction ratios were slightly more likely to be reached by rural than urban sites (small rural 92.9% vs. 91.2% urban). Mortality and transplant rates showed a more complex picture, however. Relative to urban Hispanic patients, rural Hispanic patients had elevated mortality rates both before (OR=1.25, 95%CI=1.14-1.36) and after adjustment (OR=1.11, 95%CI=1.01-1.22). Rural white non-Hispanics and blacks had lower mortality than urban white non-Hispanics and blacks, respectively, but only after adjustment. Transplant rates were lowest among black patients regardless of where they lived, with residents of small rural areas more disadvantaged than residents of urban areas (OR=0.89, 95%CI=0.82-0.96). In contrast, rural Native Americans living in remote areas were actually more likely than Native Americans living in urban areas to get a transplant (OR=1.27, 95%CI=1.01-1.59). A similar rural advantage was evident for non-Hispanic whites (OR=1.11, 95%CI=1.06-1.16).

## Summary

There were no consistent differences between rural and urban areas in diabetes treatment quality measures, and two of the largest, moderate to high quality studies found no differences. Whether rural-urban differences in diabetes care varies across regions of the country requires further exploration.[51] For all patients, having access to a physician, and possibly an endocrinologist, may increase the odds of both illness detection and adherence to treatment guidelines. The increased use of Rural Health Clinics in underserved areas has greatly improved treatment access and, consequently, adherence to treatment guidelines.[52]

There was also little evidence for a disparity between rural and urban patients with diabetes in terms of diabetes complications or the prevalence of ESRD. Once a patient had ESRD, racial differences clearly affected outcomes, and this variation across race/ethnicity groups interacted with rural vs. urban residential categories. For example, a high quality study reported that blacks with ESRD had lower transplant rates regardless of where they lived, but were more disadvantaged in rural areas.[44] In contrast, rural Native Americans were actually more likely than their urban counterparts to receive a transplant.[44]

**Table 5. Confidence Scores for Diabetes and End-Stage Renal Disease Studies**

| Study | Andrus 2004[47] | Weingar-ten 2006[41] | Krisha 2010[45] | Rosenblatt 2001[50] | Morden 2010[49] | Koopman 2006[48] | Ward 2009[46] | O'Hare 2006[44] |
|---|---|---|---|---|---|---|---|---|
| **Internal Validity** | F | F | G | F | G | F | F | G |
| Sampling Method/Bias | F | F | G | F | G | G | F | G |
| Predictors/Confounders | P | P | G | F | G | G | F | G |
| Outcomes | G | G | G | F | G | G | F | G |
| Statistical Methods | P | G | G | F | G | F | P | G |
| **External Validity** | F/P | F | F | F | F | F | F | G |
| Use of proxy variables or aggregate measures | F | F | G | G | G | G | F | G |
| Representativeness of sample (size, composition) | P | P | F | F | G | F | F | G |
| Is the study design appropriate for the research question? | F | F | F | G | F | G | F | G |
| **Overall Confidence Score** | VL | L | H/M | M | H/M | M | L | H |

## CARDIOVASCULAR DISEASE (Table 6 and Appendix C, Table 5)

Only five studies examined outpatient management of cardiovascular disease, and two of these were smaller regional studies. The largest study, and the only one for which we had at least a moderate to high Confidence Score, was done by Morden et al., (2010) on 23,780 veterans with hypertension, about one-third of whom also had a mental disorder.[49] No differences in blood pressure (BP) control were found across three RUCA categories.

A Colorado study compared quality of care for hypertension among 780 rural and urban patients with diabetes from 26 primary care sites.[53] The study relied on provider post-appointment surveys. They found that rural patients had lower systolic and diastolic BP, but that urban providers were more likely to take action than rural providers if the patient's BP were poorly controlled (39.1% vs. 27.5%, p<0.02). However, of the factors that predicted whether action was taken at a given medical visit, the number of prescribed medications and whether the patient's BP was at or near goal were the only significant predictors, possibly reflecting differences in subsample characteristics. Of note, number of prescribed medications was significantly associated with rural residence (e.g., 39% of rural residents were taking 8 or more medications, whereas only 28% of urban residents took as many; p<0.025).

The remaining studies were given fairly low Confidence Scores, and so shall be reviewed only briefly. In a study by King (2006), rural site of health care was associated with better BP control in a chart review study looking at 300 people from three separate practices in South Carolina (OR=0.3, 95%CI=0.16-0.55).[54] We rated this study as having lower quality because of the small non-random sample, lack of control of within site clustering, and use of chart indications of adherence. A second regional study, comparing one urban with one rural site in New Mexico examined differences in treatment via chart review of 200 patients, 100 with cardiovascular disease and 100 without.[55] They found that patients treated in the urban, university associated center were much more likely to receive beta-blockers or calcium channel blockers, antiplatelet therapy, and statins, and that urban patients were better at attaining BP goals (53% vs. 37%, p=0.02). LDL goals, on the other hand, were comparable in rural and urban areas (51% vs. 57%, ns). Confidence in this study's findings were considered to be low due to the sampling method, statistical approach, and variable outcome measures.

Finally, a series of case reports examined change in medication regimens in 32 elderly cardiac patients post-discharge.[56] Urban cardiac patients reported greater fluctuations in medication regimen, as suggested by the number of changes in the types of drug used after discharge compared to rural cardiac patients; however, the urban cardiac patients had worse outcomes than the rural patients despite comparable levels of cardiac disease.

## Summary

Three of the five studies reviewed were quite small, and only one study had a higher Confidence Score. That study, conducted on veterans, found no differences between rural and urban patients in control of hypertension. The Colorado study found different degrees of blood pressure control between urban and rural residents, but no differences in quality of care. However, that study consisted of patients with diabetes and had some significant flaws that compromised the reliability of the findings. The remaining studies were not of sufficient quality to draw conclusions beyond the clinics from which their samples were drawn.

**Table 6. Confidence Scores for Cardiovascular Disease Studies**

| Study | Morden 2010[49] | King 2006[54] | Colleran 2007[55] | Hicks 2010[53] | Dellasega 1999[56] |
|---|---|---|---|---|---|
| **Internal Validity** | G | P | F | F | P |
| Sampling Method/Bias | G | P | G | F | P |
| Predictors/Confounders | G | G | F | F | F |
| Outcomes | G | P | G | G | F |
| Statistical Methods | G | F | F/P | G | P |
| **External Validity** | F | P | F | F | P |
| Use of proxy variables or aggregate measures | G | P | F | G | F |
| Representativeness of sample | G | P | P | F | P |
| Study design appropriate for the research question? | F | F | G | F | P |
| **Overall Confidence Score** | H/M | VL | L | M | VL |

## HIV/AIDS (Table 7 and Appendix C, Table 6)

There were four papers that reported rural-urban differences in HIV/AIDS patients.[57-60]

In a study of 308 women from Georgia diagnosed with AIDS by 1990, non-metropolitan residence was associated with a shorter median survival time (296 days vs. 400 days for urban residence) and a lower odds of surviving 90 days (0.84 urban vs. 0.69 non-metropolitan).[57] Our confidence in the study is very low, however, given significant methodologic problems and the use of data that covered cases diagnosed over 20 years ago.

The frequency of visits per year did not differ between urban and rural residents in either adjusted or unadjusted analyses of a large observational cohort study of HIV patients in North Carolina.[59] However, all patients received care at the University of North Carolina HIV Outpatient Clinic, suggesting that distance to clinic was not a significant barrier to care. Relatedly, a national study using the HIV Cost and Services Utilization Study (HCSUS) from 1996 found that nearly three-quarters of rural HIV patients receive their HIV-related care in urban areas.[60] Only older age was associated with receiving HIV-related care in a rural setting. In contrast to the North Carolina study, nearly one-third who received their care in urban settings reported that the distance deterred them from needed clinic appointments; however, actual number of clinic appointments was not assessed. Using the same dataset, Cohn (2001) found that rural HIV-related care was more likely to be of lower quality than urban care. Specifically, they found that 73% of urban residents received highly active antiretroviral therapy (HAART) vs. only 57% of rural residents (p<0.001).[58] After adjusting for CD4 counts and the covariates (see table), urban patients had a three-fold higher odds of receiving HAART than rural patients. Moreover, whereas 75% of urban patient received prophylactic medication for *pneumocystis carinii* pneumonia, only 60% of rural residents did (p<0.007). Although not directly related to treatment variables, these differences may be due to the fact that 38% of rural patients received care from providers with little experience treating HIV patients compared to only 3% of urban residents.

## Summary

The very sparse data on the treatment of HIV/AIDS suggests that rural residents might not receive care comparable to that received by HIV infected residents living in urban areas if they receive care locally rather than travel to specialty HIV clinics in urban areas. However, no firm conclusions can be drawn from this minimal evidence base. A more recent assessment of the quality of HIV care is warranted given that diffusion of knowledge regarding treatment standards for HIV/AIDS may have occurred in the intervening period.

**Table 7. Confidence Scores for HIV/AIDS Studies**

| Study | Whyte 1992[57] | Napravnik 2006[59] | Schur 2002[60] | Cohn 2001[58] |
|---|---|---|---|---|
| **Internal Validity** | F | G/F | F | G |
| Sampling Method/Bias | G | F | G/F | G |
| Predictors/Confounders | P | G | G | G |
| Outcomes | G | G | F | G |
| Statistical Methods | F | G | G | G |
| **External Validity** | P | F | F | G/F |
| Use of proxy variables or aggregate measures | F | F | F | G |
| Representativeness of sample | P | F | F | G |
| Study design appropriate for the research question? | P | G | F | F |
| **Overall Confidence Score** | VL | M | M | H/M |

# NEUROLOGIC CONDITIONS (Table 8 and Appendix C, Table 7)

There were only three studies that examined urban/rural differences in health care for patients with multiple sclerosis (MS), and all three of them were from the same research group and were based on the same dataset. The studies were based on a survey of national MS Society members, with sampling stratified to achieve 500 MS patients in each of three population density categories: urban, within 50 miles of urban area, and more than 50 miles. Their overall response rate was a low 31%, and several aspects of the methodology resulted in our giving all three studies low Confidence Scores.[61-63] In bivariate analyses, more MS patients in rural areas had a primary progressive form of MS, but fewer reported that they were being treated with disease modifying medications (urban 64%, adjacent rural 57%, remote rural 55%).[61] More MS patients in urban areas saw a neurologist in the previous year (urban 75.4%, adjacent rural 71%, remote rural 66.5%) and more patients in remote and adjacent rural areas indicated that they had wanted to have seen a neurologist in the previous year but did not do so (urban 9.4%, adjacent rural 18.9%, remote rural 26.9%).[62] Finally, the primary reason reported for not seeking treatment was a lack of availability of mental health providers (urban 5%, adjacent rural 33%, and 13% remote rural).[63]

There were only two studies that focused on services for those who incurred a traumatic brain injury (TBI).[64,65]

A survey of 292 residents with TBI 12-18 months previously, in the Iowa Central Registry for Brain and Spinal Cord Injuries in 1998, examined self-rated health and dependence on others.[64] There were no differences between rural vs. urban areas in the association between perceived need for care and actual receipt of services; however, the authors did not examine the odds of service receipt in a multivariate model, and we rated this study with a low Confidence Score.

Two studies examined the availability of health professionals who provide the interdisciplinary care needed by those who had TBIs. A survey of health providers in Missouri in 1999 found that although nearly one-third of state residents live in rural areas, much lower percentages of all provider types related to the treatment of patients with TBIs (e.g., physiatrists, other physicians, rehab therapists, mental health providers) worked in rural areas.[65] A similar pattern was found in a nationwide study of numbers of rehabilitation therapists (physical therapists, occupational therapists, and speech-language pathologists) in counties or "county sets" in most of the contiguous United States between 1980-2000.[66] Fewer rehabilitation therapists per 100,000 residents were found in primary care health professional shortage areas. Although the number of all three types of rehabilitation therapists increased in both urban and rural county sets during the 20 year time period, the difference in the ratio of therapists per 100,000 residents remained significantly different between urban and rural areas (urban: rural rates per 100,000 for physical therapists 50.9: 35.5, occupational therapists 24.7: 15.3, and speech pathologists 35.0: 29.5).

## Summary

Findings from the three studies of rural treatment for MS, all based on the same dataset, were inconclusive given several methodologic problems with the research design, measures and analyses.

There was only one study that looked at outcomes for patients with a history of TBI in rural vs. urban settings of Iowa, but we had little confidence in the findings of that study. Two studies examining the availability of rehabilitation specialists found a paucity of such providers in many rural areas relative to urban areas. Significantly more research should be done on the course of recovery of rural TBI patients after their acute treatment, and to ascertain what types of services they receive by commuting to urban areas, what services are precluded by limited provider availability and/or travel distance, and what the impact of provider availability is on health outcomes.

**Table 8. Confidence Scores for Neurologic Conditions Studies**

| Study | Buchanan 2006a[61] | Buchanan 2006b[62] | Buchanan 2006c[63] | Schoot- man 1999[64] | Johnstone 2002[65] | Wilson 2009[66] |
|---|---|---|---|---|---|---|
| **Internal Validity** | F | F/P | F/P | F | G | G |
| Sampling Method/Bias | P | P | P | G | G | G |
| Predictors/Confounders | G | G | G | F | G | G |
| Outcomes | F | F | F | F | G | G |
| Statistical Methods | P | P | P | F | G | G |
| **External Validity** | F/P | F/P | F/P | F | G/F | G/F |
| Use of proxy variables or aggregate measures | F | F | F | F | F | F |
| Representativeness of sample | P | P | P | F | G | G |
| Study design appropriate for the research question? | F | P | P | F | G | G |
| **Overall Confidence Score** | L/VL | VL | VL | L | H/M | H/M |

## MENTAL HEALTH (Table 9 and Appendix C, Table 8)

There were three studies that compared suicide rates and medication use between rural and urban areas,[67-69] two studies that examined the odds of hospitalization,[70,71] five papers that addressed MH service access among rural residents with severe mental illness,[72-76] three studies that examined rural-urban differences in treatment of mood disorders,[69,77,78] one study examining PTSD,[79] five studies that examined receipt of alcohol/drug treatment,[80-84] and four papers that examined whether subgroups of rural residents were less likely to get mental health treatment.[85-88]

A large national study of suicide completers found an association between suicide and antidepressant prescription rates.[67] In rural areas, the suicide rates were higher than in urban areas (17.14 per 100,000 in the most rural vs. 11.51 per 100,000 in the most urban). Within these rural areas, there were fewer prescriptions for antidepressants and, of those that were written, a higher proportion of them were for the older tricyclic antidepressants (ratios of tricyclics vs. newer antidepressants were 1:1 in rural vs. 1:2 in urban). Only prescriptions for non-tricyclic antidepressants were associated with reduced suicide rates. A second study examining suicide rates among 41 county clusters in California from 1993-2001, found similar elevations in suicide rates among rural counties, but no association between suicide rates and the availability of either health care providers or physicians.[68] Although suggestive, these studies use only aggregate measures and limited control for confounders, resulting in lower Confidence Scores. One study that followed 470 depressed people in Arkansas found no difference in the odds or quality of depression treatment between rural and urban residents, but did find an elevated rate of suicide attempts among those in rural areas.[69]

Both studies that examined hospitalization rates per county for major mental illnesses used the 2000 Health Care Cost and Utilization Project database for 14 states.[70,71] Both studies reported similar findings – that rural areas had lower hospitalization rates. Specifically, hospitalization rates for schizophrenia were greatest in the most urban areas relative to all others ($p<0.05$).[71] Similarly, hospitalizations for depression were lower in rural vs. more urban areas (e.g., 49% lower in the most rural counties, $p<0.05$).[70] No relationship was found between provider availability and hospitalization rates for schizophrenia, but positive relationships were found between availability of physicians and hospitals and hospitalization rates for depression ($p<0.05$); however, there was no relationship between hospitalization rates and availability of psychiatrists.[71] Both studies examined environmental predictors of hospitalization rates and found that factors associated with urban living (e.g., housing stress) were predictive of higher rates, where as rural factors (e.g., farm-based economies) appeared to be protective. Because the base rates of mental illness in the counties studied were not known a priori and because both studies relied on aggregate measures, it cannot be determined from these studies whether urban environmental factors are conducive to the development or exacerbation of mental illness (or highly rural areas protective), or whether mentally ill people are more likely to migrate to urban areas. Consequently, our Confidence Scores are lower for these studies.

There were five articles that addressed accessibility of MH services for rural residents with severe mental illness, one of which was an examination of the VA's mental health intensive case management program (MHICM). Three of these focused on whether rural residents with serious mental illness had difficulty accessing needed services, one examined whether travel time affected the number of mental health treatment appointments, whereas the fifth examined access within the context of continuity of care.

Rost et al. (1998) screened 11,078 adults in Arkansas for mental illness and compared rural-urban differences in a very small subsample with bipolar disorder (29 rural and 24 urban residents) on service utilization and outcomes.[46] Rural residents were much more likely to be seen only in a general medical setting (OR=22.1, 95%CI=2.5-198.3), to have needed acute medical or mental health care (OR=5.8, 95%CI=0.8-40.7), and to have experienced a manic episode in the year following the baseline assessment (OR=4.0, 95%CI=0.8-20.5). Although the screened sample was large, the resulting small number of those with bipolar disorder resulted in a low Confidence Score rating. The same study produced a larger number of patients with major depression, but only n=106 were included in a study examining the relationship between travel time to a preferred provider, number of depression-related appointments, and the odds of receiving guideline concordant depression treatment.[74] Distance from a preferred provider was significantly associated with a reduced number of visits in adjusted analyses ($p<0.05$). Increased travel time, in turn, was associated with reduced odds of guideline concordant treatment (OR=0.292, CI= 0.087-0.987).

A study of 258 patients with schizophrenia seen in public mental health settings (primarily VA) in Arkansas between 1992-1999, found that rural residence was associated with an increased risk of an irregular vs. regular pattern of mental health service use in adjusted analyses (OR=1.99, 95%CI=1.07-3.71).[73] For all patients, comorbid substance abuse increased the odds of infrequent or irregular mental health service use. However, among rural residents, the negative impact of comorbid substance abuse was significant only if the patient did not have contact with their family at least once per week (OR=41.94 for infrequent service use vs. regular MH use among those with minimal family contact). This suggests that the role of family in managing patients with severe mental illness may differ in rural vs. urban areas.

The VA study of the amount and types of care received by 5,221 patients with serious mental illness enrolled in a MHICM program reported that patients in rural areas received fewer types of services than urban patients.[75] Although the difference in patient contact between rural and urban residents differed only slightly (though significantly), rural residents were less likely to receive several types of recovery-related services, such as psychotherapy (83% urban vs. 67% isolated rural), substance abuse treatment (35% urban vs. 29% rural town and 12% isolated rural), and rehab services (48% urban vs. 42% rural towns and 27% isolated rural) despite comparable symptomatology. Moreover, rural residents were more likely to be seen by only one person on the treatment team than urban patients. Whether this affected recovery is unclear, as all symptom measures were assessed at the time of program enrollment.

The fourth study focused on the ease of care transition from inpatient to outpatient services for 4,930 patients with serious mental illness who were discharged from Virginia state hospitals in 1992.[72] Specifically, they found that rural residents had significantly better continuity of care than urban patients in that the community mental health centers associated with outpatient treatment for rural residents were much more likely to have copies of the discharge records (89% rural vs. 76% urban), to have contacted the patient during the hospitalization (58% rural vs. 49% urban), to have made contact with the patient after discharge (82% rural vs. 78% urban), and to have seen the patient for an appointment (79% rural vs. 76% urban). Despite some limitations in rural mental health services for those with serious mental illness, the smaller size of rural community mental health clinics likely contributed to the post-discharge continuity. Of note, there were no differences in a composite of these continuity measures between black and white patients in rural areas, but in urban areas, blacks were clearly disadvantaged. That is, race disparities existed mostly in urban areas.

There were two other studies that used the same dataset that examined rural-urban differences in treatment of bipolar disorder referenced above, and these subsequent studies focused on Arkansans who screened positive for major depression. Examining quality of care and outcomes for the 434 who met criteria for major depression, Rost (1999) reported that there were no rural-urban differences in the odds of outpatient treatment of depression, type of care, odds of care meeting clinical guidelines for acute stage treatment, or adherence to treatment.[77] Urban residents were more likely to have been high users of specialty mental health care, with 22% making 23 or more visits during the follow-up year compared to 4% of rural residents (p=0.04). Rural residents, were significantly more likely to be hospitalized for physical problems (OR=3.05, 95%CI=1.23-7.53). In the second paper, the odds of these elevated admissions were really significant only during the first 6 months after baseline, with rural residents having much higher odds of hospitalization for physical (6.1% vs. 0.3%, p<0.01) and mental health (9.8% vs. 1.1%, p<0.05) problems.[69]

Rural vs. urban hospitalization rates for depressed patients was also examined in a secondary analysis of two separate depression treatment studies, involving 1,455 patients from 11 states.[78] As in the Arkansas study, it was found that the odds for hospitalization in a six month follow-up period were greater among rural residents for physical health problems (OR=1.8, 95%CI=1.2-2.8). At 18 months, rural residents had more hospitalizations for mental health problems (OR=2.3, 95%CI=1.0-5.4). Although there were no differences in the rate of outpatient specialty care between urban and rural residents, only about one-third of all patients in the sample indicated that they took antidepressants for at least two of the previous six months. Because of the sampling and other methodologic problems inherent in this study, however, our Confidence Score was low.

Only one very small study examined service use among patients diagnosed with PTSD.[79] No significant differences were found in the number of specialty PTSD clinic appointments between 48 urban and 52 rural veterans. The absence of a finding is inconclusive, however, given the inadequate power to detect possible differences and the limited number of confounders included in the analyses.

There were five studies that examined receipt of alcohol/drug treatment. Two studies of moderate to moderately high quality found no rural-urban differences in treatment utilization,[80,81] and three of moderate to low quality found greater treatment utilization among residents living in urban areas.[82-84]

In a Florida study of 2,222 out-of-treatment injection drug users and crack smokers, the rate of drug treatment receipt in the previous 24 months was twice as high for drug users in the urban Miami area than for drug users in the rural Immokalee area (16.3% vs. 4.4%, $p<0.001$).[82] Moreover, those in the urban Miami area who received any treatment were in treatment for twice as long as those treated in the more rural Immokalee area (28.3 weeks vs. 12.1 weeks, $p<0.001$). Importantly, however, there was a much lower rate in the Immokalee area of unsuccessful attempts at getting treatment (4.9% vs. 10.8%, $p<0.001$), suggesting that the lower rate of treatment receipt among the rural drug users was at least partially due to differences in treatment seeking. Given the sampling issues, however, the generalizability of this study is limited.

Comparable treatment rates were reported in a lower quality study by Robertson and Donnermeyer (1997),[83] who assessed rates of treatment for drug abuse in the 1991 National Household Survey on Drug Abuse. Among the 3,629 subjects included in their study, only 10.8% of the nonmetropolitan-rural respondents received drug treatment and, among those who used illegal drugs in the past 12 months, the rate dropped to 5.6% (vs. 6.6% of the remaining survey respondents). Finally, in a study examining continuity of care for 4,621 veterans discharged from inpatient alcohol treatment programs, rural residence increased the odds of attending an aftercare appointment.[84] However, distance to treatment was a significantly greater treatment barrier for rural residents than for urban residents. [84]

To better define which rural residents were less likely to utilize mental health care, there were four papers using national samples that examined whether subgroups of rural residents were particularly unlikely or disadvantaged. Using data from two panels of the MEPS between 1996-1998, Petterson (2003) observed that rural residents who received mental health care had fewer visits per calendar year than urban residents ($p<0.01$), had higher rates of hospitalization ($p<0.04$), and were more likely to only see a physician for their treatment ($p<0.02$).[85] Rural residents had fewer mental health visits even after adjustment for demographic factors ($p<0.01$). After adjustments were made for income, insurance and physical health status in addition to demographic variables, the differences between rural and urban residents in mental health care use were only a trend ($p<0.1$), suggesting that differences in access accounted for much of the observed disparity for rural residents. Importantly, Petterson (2003) noted that urban residents who reported only "fair mental health" were nearly twice as likely as similarly rated rural residents to have sought mental health care (38% vs. 24%, p<0.01) suggesting that rural and urban residents may also differ in perceived need for care. [85]

In a separate study, Petterson (2009) used four panels from the same database (representing 1996-2000) to examine whether rural-urban differences observed in the 2003 study were similar across racial/ethnic groups.[86] They observed a rural disadvantage for receipt of any mental health treatment among whites, with 9.4% in urban areas having received mental health care but only 7.3% of those in the most rural areas. Both blacks and Hispanics were less likely to receive any mental health care or specialty mental health care regardless of whether they lived in a rural or urban area. However, whereas the difference between blacks and non-Hispanic whites was significant independent of residence urbanicity, the disparity between blacks and whites was greater in urban areas than in rural areas (urban OR=0.41, 95%CI=0.35-0.49; rural OR=0.58, 95%CI=0.35-0.94). The same pattern was seen when only specialty mental health care was considered -- the difference between blacks and whites was significantly different in urban areas, but not in the most rural areas (urban OR=0.43, 95%CI=0.36-0.53; rural OR=0.62, 95%CI=0.28-1.39). Differences between whites and Hispanics follow a similar pattern except that specialty mental health care differed only in urban areas, whereas the receipt of "any mental health care" differed in urban and larger rural areas but not in the most rural areas.

Another study using the same dataset (MEPS from 1996-2000) focused on gender differences in mental health care use between rural and urban residents.[87] Women from any geographic area were significantly more likely to have had any mental health treatment or specialty mental health treatment than men (10% vs. 5.8% and 6.3% vs. 3.8%; p<0.01). They found that both men and women in rural areas were less likely to receive specialty mental health services relative to their urban counterparts even after adjustment for demographics, insurance and usual source of care (women urban-rural OR=1.52, men urban-rural OR=1.94; p<0.05).

In examining mental health treatment across disorders, the National Comorbidity Study-Replication study conducted between 2001-2003,[88] found that urban residents were much more likely to have received mental health services within the previous 12 months than rural residents (urban vs. rural OR=2.1, 95%CI=1.7-2.7), and more likely to have received specialty mental health treatment (urban vs. rural OR=2.2, 95%CI=1.2-4.1). However, treatment adequacy from mental health specialists (but not general medical providers) when it did occur, was found to be lower in urban areas among those who received any mental health treatment (urban vs. rural OR=0.4, 95%CI=0.2-0.8).

## Summary

Many studies of mental health services in rural vs. urban areas focused on specific regions, which may not be generalizable to other parts of the country. Most studies examined differences in service provision and only a few associated any differences that were found with patient outcomes. This limited the conclusions that could be drawn regarding the adequacy of rural vs. urban health care. In those few studies that assessed patient outcomes, no consistent evidence for a rural disadvantage was found. Moreover, while rural residents were found to receive fewer MH services than urban residents in several studies, the clinical impact of this difference was not assessed.

Two studies that focused on the relationship between suicide and mental health care parameters used aggregate (i.e., county) measures for both variables. Although the elevated suicide rates could suggest differences in health care access and/or quality, it is unclear whether the observed association between reduced county mental health care parameters (e.g., new generation antidepressant use) and suicide rate would remain if the individual (vs. the county) were the unit of analysis. One prospective study found elevated suicide rates among depressed rural residents in Arkansas, but the small numbers made it impossible to determine if this were related to differences in mental health care.

Of note, two studies found greater racial disparities in mental health treatment receipt in urban areas. This could reflect a selectively improved access for whites in urban areas or a greater difficulty with access for minorities. Moreover, it also underscores the importance of examining race-rurality interactions, since ignoring such interactions could result in both race and/or rural disparities being attenuated.

## PROCESSES OR STRUCTURE OF CARE (APPENDIX C, TABLES 9-13)

There were a number of studies that compared various aspects of health care structure or processes between urban and rural health care settings without focusing on either a particular medical or mental health condition or, in most cases, without reference to health outcomes. We review these studies here as they relate to Key Question #2.

### Use of Medication (Appendix C, Table 9)

There were a number of studies that examined the use of prescription medications without associating medication use with health outcomes. The studies on medication use examined prevalence and/or intensity of medication use,[56,89-94] expenditures for prescription drugs,[92,93,95] likelihood of having a usual pharmacy,[94] and degree of change in postdischarge medication regimen.[56] All of the study samples consisted of outpatients over 65 years old. Three studies[92,93,95] used national samples and the rest used samples from a single state. Two of the studies[92,95] that had used a national sample had relatively small sample sizes ($N<1,100$). The sample sizes for the single-state studies varied widely, ranging from 32[56] to 18,641.[91] One study was of moderate quality, three were of low to moderate quality, and four were of low quality.

Of the seven studies that examined prevalence and/or intensity of medication use, all but one were rated with moderate to low Confidence Scores. Among these studies, five reported significant rural-urban differences on the number of medications used; however, the direction of effects was inconsistent. Comparing the number of medications prescribed for cardiac patients discharged from a tertiary hospital, Dellasega et al. (1999) found a greater number of drugs prescribed over time for urban patients than for rural patients (e.g., 5.9 vs. 4.2 for urban and rural, respectively, at four weeks post-discharge), even after controlling for severity of illness at time of discharge.[56] Similarly, Hanlon et al. (1996) found greater use of prescription drugs among urban elderly residents than their rural counterparts (OR=1.40, 95% 95%CI 1.18-2.04).[90] Mueller and Schur (2004), on the other hand, found greater number of prescriptions filled by elderly rural Medicare beneficiaries compared to elderly urban beneficiaries (for those with drug coverage, medians of 23 and 20.8, p<0.01, for rural and urban, respectively; for those without drug coverage, medians of 18.1 and 16.0, p<0.05, for rural and urban, respectively).[93] Notably, rural residents were somewhat less likely to have coverage for prescription drugs (59.4% rural vs. 75.4% urban, p<0.01).

Rural vs. Urban Ambulatory Health Care: A Systematic Review

Evidence-based Synthesis Program

**Table 9. Confidence Scores for Mental Health Studies**

| Study | Gibbons 2005[67] | Fiske 2005[68] | Farrell 1996[72] | Fischer 2008[73] | Mohamed 2009[75] | Rost & Owen 1998[76] | Rost 1999[77] | Fortney 1999[74] | Fortney 2007[70] | Fortney 2009[71] | Rost & Zhang 1998[69] | Rost 2007[78] | Elhai 2004[79] | Booth 2000[80] | Grant 1996[81] | Metsch 1999[82] | Fortney 1995[84] | Robertson 1997[83] | Petterson 2003[85] | Petterson 2009[86] | Hauenstein 2006[87] | Wang 2005[88] |
|---|---|---|---|---|---|---|---|---|---|---|---|---|---|---|---|---|---|---|---|---|---|---|
| **Internal Validity** | | | | | | | | | | | | | | | | | | | | | | |
| Sampling Method/Bias | G | G | G | G | G | G | G | G | G | G | G | F | G | G | G | F | G | G | G | G | G | G |
| Predictors/Confounders | F | F | P | F | G | F | G | G | F | F | G | G | P | G | G/F | G | G | F | F | G | G | G |
| Outcomes | G | G | G | F | F | G | G | F | G | G | G | F | G | G | G | G | G | F | G | F | F | G |
| Statistical Methods | G | F | F | G | F | G | G | G | G | G | G | G/F | F | G | G | F | G | F | F | G | G | G |
| **External Validity** | F/P | F/P | F | F | F | F | F | F | F | F | F | F | P | G/F | F | F | F | F | F | F | F | F |
| Use of proxy variables or aggregate measures | P | P | G | G | G | G | F | G | F | F | F | F | G | F | F/P | G | F | F | F | F | F | G |
| Representativeness of sample | G | G | G | F | G | P | G/F | F/P | G | G | G/F | F | F/P | G | G | P | G | G/F | G | G | G | F |
| Study design appropriate for the research question? | F | F | F | G | F | F | G | F | F | F | G | F/P | P | G | G/F | F | F | F/P | G | G | G | G |
| **Overall Confidence Score** | L | L | M | M | M | L | M | M/L | M/L | M/L | M | L | VL | H/M | M | M/L | M | L | M | M | M | H/M |

In a study of non-cognitively impaired residents 65 years and older in western Texas, Xu et al. (2003) found no difference in the odds of prescription drug use between individuals living in urban counties and those living in rural counties (i.e., counties outside of MSA or with a population less than 50,000); however, those living in frontier counties (i.e., counties with fewer than 7 people per square mile) had lower odds (OR=0.59, $p<0.01$) of prescription medication receipt.[94]

In contrast to these findings from lower quality studies, a large study of 18,641 Pennsylvania residents by Lago et al, (1993) did not find a rural-urban difference in medical claims for the number of prescriptions.[91] Other studies using national samples similarly found no rural-urban difference in drug expenditures between rural and urban residents.[92,93] Some support was found for a race by population density interaction for medication use in a study of 4,163 residents in North Carolina.[89] Specifically, urban whites were more likely to take greater number of prescription drugs than rural whites ($\beta$=0.21, $SE$=0.10, p<0.05), but there was no association between rurality and intensity of prescription drug use among blacks ($\beta$=0.12, $SE$=0.08, $ns$). A secondary analysis of data from a national survey of 996 elderly participants also failed to find rural-urban differences in the percentage of family income spent on drugs after controlling for income, insurance, and health status.[95]

The odds of having a usual pharmacy were lower for frontier county residents compared to urban residents in West Texas (OR=0.64, p<0.01), but rural residents were more likely to report that their pharmacies provided medication delivery services.[94]

## Medical Procedures and Diagnostic Tests (Appendix C, Table 10)

Two studies, both of which received low Confidence Scores, looked at use of medical procedures or diagnostic tests. Miller (1995) examined use of medical procedures and services provided by physicians among rural and urban Medicare beneficiaries.[96] The use of most services, including office visits and consultations, imaging services, and diagnostic testing, were found to be lower in rural areas compared to urban areas. Focusing on racial disparities in service utilization, Escarce et al. (1993) compared use of 32 medical procedures between white and black patients living in urban and rural areas.[97] The results showed an interaction of rurality and race on 8 (or 57%) of 14 outpatient medical procedures, with racial disparities being greater in rural than in urban areas.

## Medical Appointments with Providers (Appendix C, Table 11)

Findings were mixed across 10 studies (1 of high quality, 5 of moderate quality, 2 of low to moderate quality, and 2 of low quality) examining frequency of ambulatory care visits. While four studies found no differences in visit frequency between rural and urban,[29,98-100] four studies found that number of appointments tended to increase as population density increased.[8,101-103] Based on data from the 1984 National Health Interview Survey on people 65 yr and older, it was found that those who lived in non-metropolitan areas were 35% less likely than non-inner city metropolitan residents to visit a physician. Using a more recent cohort of that database (1992) and focusing on the 112,246 residents under 65 yr, Mueller and colleagues (1998) found that rural residents as a group were less likely to have seen a physician in the previous 12 months.[103] Minority status and living in the Southern part of the US were independent predictors of not seeing a physician in the previous 12 months; however, the strongest predictor was a lack of insurance (OR=0.42, 95%CI=0.40-0.44). In a national study of any health care use in the past 12 months among 50,993 respondents to the National Health Interview Surveys from 1999-2000, 78% of urban residents and

79% of rural residents reported using at least some health care.[100] Similar findings were reported by a second national study using the Medical Expenditures Panel Survey from 1996 which found no difference across rural or urban areas in the odds of having at least one ambulatory visit in the past year.[102] However, rural residents reported fewer visits on average than residents of large metropolitan (4.9 visits vs. 6.1 visits, p<0.02). For individuals with at least one visit, the number of visits ranged from 6.5 for rural residents to 8.3 for large metropolitan residents (p<0.001).

Weeks et al. (2005) examined the number of primary, specialty, and mental health visits from 1997-1999 among rural vs. urban veterans 65 years and older living in New England.[8] Rural veterans had fewer visits in all three treatment sectors. A study comparing 25,092 veterans at 108 community-based outpatient clinics (CBOCs) with 26,936 veterans at 72 VA medical centers (VAMCs) found more primary care visits (difference=0.10 visits) but fewer specialty care visits (difference=-1.42) per year among CBOC patients compared to VAMC patients.[104] The same pattern of results was found an earlier study that used smaller samples of CBOCs and VAMCs.[105]

## Usual Source of Care (Appendix C, Table 12)

We identified seven cross-sectional studies (two of moderate quality, three of low to moderate quality, and two of low quality) that addressed issues related to having a usual source of care (i.e., a specific clinic from which they receive care). Four of the studies included nationwide samples of patients with sample sizes ranging from 3,871 to 50,993.[48,100,102,106] Three of the studies were regional, specifically west Texas[107,108] and North Carolina.[98] Sample sizes in these studies ranged from 2,097 to 4,162. One of the studies included only active duty, uniformed service members.[106] Three studies included only patients age 65 and older,[98,107,108] and one study included only patients 18 to 64 years of age.[100] There was one study that compared only individuals of Hispanic or non-Hispanic white race/ethnicity.[107] Overall, we found that similar percentages of rural and urban residents report having a usual source of care. The percentages of rural and urban residents who reported having had a health care visit in the past year similarly did not differ by geographic location.

Six studies specifically looked at whether individuals had a usual source of care. In a large nationwide survey of individuals ages 18-64 years, 82% of urban respondents and 83% of rural respondents reported having a usual source of care.[100] Although there was no difference in the odds of having a usual source of care between respondents from urban and rural areas, race/ethnicity differences were found (e.g., 68% of Hispanics vs. 85% of whites reported a usual source of care) and these disparities were comparable in urban and rural areas.[100] Koopman (2006), using the National Health and Nutrition Examination Survey from 1988-1994, also found that Urban Hispanics were more likely than either urban or rural whites or rural Hispanics to report a lack of usual source of health care (11.4% vs. 1.8% urban whites, 6.5% rural whites, and 5.1% rural Hispanics; p<0.01).[48]

 In another national study with a similar patient population, the percentages of patients who reported having a usual source of care were 87% in the most rural counties, 89% in counties adjacent to a large metropolitan areas, 78% in large metropolitan counties, and 78% in smaller metropolitan counties.[102] In the adjusted model, patients in the most rural areas and those in rural areas adjacent to large metropolitan areas were more likely to have a usual source of care than residents in large metropolitan areas. Other factors significantly associated with having a usual source of care included worse health and higher income.

Two regional studies of patients over 64 years old found that between 94% and 96% reported having a usual source of care with no difference between urban and rural residents[98,108] In the adjusted model, having insurance other than Medicare/Medicaid was associated with increased odds of having a usual source of care while Hispanic ethnicity was associated with decreased odds.[108] Both studies also looked at whether the respondent had a personal provider. No differences were found between rural and urban areas in the odds of having a personal provider (87%).[108] Hispanic ethnicity and lower income were associated with decreased odds.[108] The second study reported a rural advantage for continuity of care with a primary care provider (88% rural vs. 82% urban; p<0.05).[98] A third study, comparing Hispanic and non-Hispanic whites in rural or frontier counties of west Texas reported that the likelihood of having a personal provider was not associated with degree of rurality; however, non-Hispanic whites were significantly more likely to report that they consulted their personal doctor or nurse.[107]

Three studies reported results related to ability to obtain care.[98,106,107] A nationwide survey of over 3,800 Department of Defense beneficiaries found that health plans and health care, ability to get care quickly, and doctor communication were rated significantly higher by residents in areas adjacent to metropolitan areas or in non-adjacent areas. Getting needed care and customer services were rated higher by residents of metropolitan areas.[106] A study of Hispanic and non-Hispanic whites in rural and frontier areas of west Texas found lower percentages of Hispanics reporting that they see a specialist when needed, that they are able to obtain transportation to the doctors' office, and that they see a doctor or nurse as soon as they want for both illness/injury and routine care. In an adjusted analysis, Hispanic ethnicity was no longer associated with decreased ability to obtain care but remained significantly associated with decreased ability to see a doctor or nurse when they wanted to. Residence in a frontier or rural county was not related to ability to obtain care or to obtain care without a long wait.[98] Finally, in a study of 4,162 residents of urban or rural counties in North Carolina, 6% of the urban respondents and 10% of the rural respondents (a non-significant difference) reported that they put off care due to transportation difficulties while14% of urban and 25% of rural respondents put off care due to the cost (p<0.05).[98]

## Provider Availability and Expertise (Appendix C, Table 13)

We identified 12 cross-sectional studies related to provider availability and expertise. Four studies were national studies.[28,66,109,110] One study was conducted in eight states in southeastern United States.[111] One study included clinicians from California and Washington.[112] The remaining studies were conducted in Wisconsin,[113] Texas,[114] Florida,[115,116] Washington,[117] or Georgia.[118] Three studies enrolled patients,[110,111,113] seven studies enrolled providers,[28,109,112,115-118] and two studies presented data by county.[66,114] Two of the studies were of high quality, five were of low to moderate quality, and five were of low quality. Overall, the evidence suggests that more remote locations are underserved by health care providers. People who live in these areas are more likely to see a family practice physician, a physician assistant, or a nurse practitioner. In one state, services are being decreased or eliminated by both rural and urban physicians. There is limited nationwide data on this topic.

Nationwide, the availability of primary care physicians per 10,000 residents decreases in an almost linear fashion from an urban high of 17.8 (SD=16.1) to a low of 7.2 (SD=7.8) in rural areas adjacent to a micropolitan area.[28] The ratio was slightly higher in remote rural regions with a ratio of 9.2 (SD=8.9),[28] but the variability across remote regions can be highly problematic.

For example, the distribution of physicians and physician assistants was examined in rural and remote counties of Texas using the Texas Medical Board Web site and from US Census Data.[114] Seventeen of 254 Texas counties had no licensed doctors or physician assistants. Statewide, there was one physician assistant for every 13.6 physicians. In the 60 frontier counties, however, the ratio was one physician assistant for every 2.3 physicians. Frontier counties, then, have not only a diminished availability of medical providers, but more of the providers that they do have are physician extenders. Patient perceptions of physician availability were consistent with the epidemiologic assessments. Biola et al. (2009) surveyed 4,879 patients living in 150 rural counties in the southeastern United States, and examined agreement with the statement "I feel there are enough doctors in my community."[111] As would be expected, patients who lived in areas with more physicians relative to the county population were more likely to respond that there were enough physicians. Of interest, the perception that there were an insufficient number of physicians was greater not only among patients who live in areas with fewer physicians relative to county residents, but also among those who traveled more than 30 minutes for care, those who lived in a more impoverished county or who had problems with the cost of care, and among those who lacked confidence in their physician's level of expertise.

As noted previously, differences in provider availability were not only found for primary health care providers. A nationwide study of numbers of rehabilitation therapists (physical therapists, occupational therapists, and speech-language pathologists) between 1980-2000, found that although the disparity in therapist availability between rural and urban areas had improved over the 20 year period, that the ratio of therapists per 100,000 residents remained significantly different between urban and rural areas (urban:rural rates per 100,000 for physical therapists 50.9:35.5, occupational therapists 24.7:15.3, and speech pathologists 35.0:29.5).[66]

In addition to limitations in provider availability, rural residents often have different types of providers available to them. A nationwide study of over 34,000 patients from non-metropolitan areas had greater adjusted odds of receiving services from family physicians, nurse practitioners, or physician assistants and lower adjusted odds of receiving services from general internists or non-surgical specialists.[110] Similarly, in the Wisconsin Longitudinal Study,[113] primary provider type was determined among survey respondents who indicated they had a usual source of care and compared across metropolitan, micropolitan, or nonmetropolitan (i.e., rural) areas.[113] Overall, 4.5% of respondents reported that a physician assistant or nurse practitioner was their primary care provider and, in adjusted analyses, these provider types were more common among nonmetropolitan residents. Also consistent with findings was a study of over 28,000 clinicians practicing in California and over 5,600 clinicians practicing in Washington State.[112] Of physician assistants practicing in California, 22% were in rural areas. A similar pattern was observed in Washington. Family physicians, nurse practitioners, and physician assistants were more likely to practice in a rural area (relative to obstetrics/gynecology). Physician extenders in rural areas often work longer hours, see more patients and provide care to more patients without insurance than their urban counterparts.[118] Differences were found not only in the prevalence of physician extenders, but also in the type of physicians practicing in rural areas. For example, in a study of over 4,000 providers in Washington State,[117] family physicians were most likely to provide care in a rural area; psychiatrists, cardiologist, and gastroenterologists were least likely. Although the diagnostic scope of practice was similar for rural and urban physicians, rural obstetrician-gynecologists were more likely to care for diagnoses outside of their specialty and rural general surgeons were more likely to care for gastrointestinal disorders (vs. cardiac conditions for urban surgeons). Not surprisingly, procedure rates were higher for rural physicians.

Of concern is the fact that often the qualifications of physician extenders in rural areas may not be comparable to those practicing in urban settings. A survey of nurse practitioners, certified nurse midwives, and physician assistants in Georgia found that of 554 nurse practitioners who responded, 31% were working in a rural environment.[118] Rural nurse practitioners were less likely to have had a bachelor's degree and fewer had specialty credentials. This may be particularly concerning given that they were more likely to provide care in solo and clinic practice settings. Of 73 certified nurse midwives, 29% worked in a rural setting. Rural certified nurse midwives also had fewer specialty credentials, worked more hours per week, and saw more patients per hour. Of the 18% of 452 physician assistants practicing in rural settings, fewer had at least a bachelor's degree compared to those practicing in urban settings. Although there is limited data comparing the quality of care between rural primary care providers who are physician extenders and those who are physicians, patients in the Wisconsin Longitudinal Study whose usual source of care was a physician assistant or nurse practitioner were more likely to report lower satisfaction with access to care (beta=$-0.22$, 95%CI=$-0.35$-$-0.09$), and were less likely to have received a complete health exam (OR=0.74, 95%CI = 0.55-0.99) or a mammogram (OR=0.65, 95%CI=0.45-0.93).[113.] However, a national Web survey of physician assistants in 2008 (response rate 49%), found that rural physician assistants were better at diagnosing and treating dermatologic conditions than their urban counterparts ($p<0.03$).[109] This was interpreted as being most likely due to the larger number of dermatologic cases seen by rural practitioners (78% rural see most dermatologic cases vs. 62% of urban physician assistants). Importantly, the referral rate for specialty treatment did not differ by rural-urban practice settings.

Two studies, both conducted in Florida, reported that physicians in both urban and rural area were curtailing the services that they offered, largely in response to malpractice costs.[115,116] Overall, 60% of 308 respondents from both rural and urban areas reported that "delivery of patient services in their practice had been decreased or eliminated in the last year."[116] Of the 539 respondents to a survey of rural physicians, 55% reported they decreased or eliminated patient services in the past year. Among the services decreased were mental health services (reported decreased by 35%), vaccine administration (29%), office-based surgeries (40%), Pap smears (24%), x-rays (24%), endoscopies (43%), and electrocardiograms (11%). Additionally, there was a significantly greater reduction or elimination of services, overall, by physicians who saw higher numbers of Medicare patients.[115]

## Summary

There is limited availability of any health care providers in highly rural areas, and specialists in particular. There was some weak evidence that physician extenders in rural areas may not have comparable credentials to their urban counterparts. Rural residents were more likely to have family medicine physicians as their primary care doctors, as well as primary providers who were physician extenders. Having fewer health care choices seemed to increase the odds of remaining with the same provider over time, thereby improving continuity of care. There is weak evidence that in some parts of the country, health care providers in highly rural areas may not have comparable credentials as their counterparts in urban area. It is unclear to what extent this might generalize to other areas.

Rural vs. Urban Ambulatory Health Care: A Systematic Review

Evidence-based Synthesis Program

**Table 10. Confidence Scores for Processes or Structure of Care Studies**

| Study | Dellasaga 1999[56] | Fillenbaum 1993[89] | Hanlon 1996[90] | Lago 1993[91] | Lillard 1999[92] | Mueller 2004[93] | Xu 2003[94] | Rogowski 1997[95] | Miller 1995[96] | Escarce 1993[97] | Blazer 1995[98] | McConell 1993[99] | Saag 1998[29] | Himes 1993[101] | Larson 2003[102] | Mueller 1998[103] | Weeks 2005[8] | Maciejewski 2007[104] | Fortney 2002[105] |
|---|---|---|---|---|---|---|---|---|---|---|---|---|---|---|---|---|---|---|---|
| **Internal Validity (G, F, P)** | F | G | G | F | F | F | F | F | F | F | F | F | F | F | F | F | F | G | F |
| Sampling Method/Bias | F | G | G | F | F | G | F | F | F | F | F | F | F | G | G | G | G | G | G |
| Predictors/Confounders | F | G | G | F | F | F | G | F | F | F | G | F | G | F | G | G | F | G | F |
| Outcomes | F | G | F | G | F | G | F | F | F | F | F | F | F | F | F | G | G | G | G |
| Statistical Methods | F | G | G | G | F | F | G | F | F | F | G | F | G | F | F | F | F | G | F |
| **External Validity (G, F, P)** | P | F | F | F | F | F | P | F | F | P | F | G | F | G | G | F | F | G | F |
| Use of proxy variables or aggregate measures | F | G | G | G | F | G | F | F | F | F | G | F | G | G | G | F | G | G | G |
| Representativeness of sample (size, composition) | P | F | F | F | F | G | F | F | F | F | F | F | F | G | G | G | G | G | G |
| Is the study design appropriate for the research question? | P | G | G | G | F | P | P | F | F | P | F | F | P | G | G | F | F | G | F |
| Overall Confidence Score | L | M/L | M/L | M | L | M/L | L | L | L | L | M/L | L | L | M | M | M | M | H | M |

**Table 10. Confidence Scores for Processes or Structure of Care Studies**

| Study | Meza 2006[106] | Glover 2004[100] | Borders 2004[107] | Rohrer 2004[108] | Koopman 2006[48] | Wilson 2009[66] | Ferrer 2007[110] | Biola 2009[111] | Grumbach 2003[112] | Everett 2009[113] | Jones 2008[114] | Gunderson 2006[115] | Manachemi 2006[116] | Baldwin 1999[117] | Strickland 1998[118] | Ladika 2009[28] | Brown 2009[109] |
|---|---|---|---|---|---|---|---|---|---|---|---|---|---|---|---|---|---|
| **Internal Validity (G, F, P)** | P | G | F | F | F | G | F | F | F | F | G | F | F | G | F | G | P |
| Sampling Method/Bias | P | G | F | F | G | G | F | P | F | F | G | F | F | G | F | G | P |
| Predictors/Confounders | F | G | G | G | G | N/A | F | G | F | F | N/A | N/A | N/A | N/A | N/A | N/A | F |
| Outcomes | F | G | F | F | G | G | G | P | F | G | G | F | F | G | G | G | P |
| Statistical Methods | F | G | G | G | F | G | F | G | G | G | N/A | G | G | G | G | G | F |
| **External Validity (G, F, P)** | F | F | F | F | F | G/F | F | P | F | F | G | F | F | F | F | G | P |
| Use of proxy variables or aggregate measures | G | G | G | G | G | F | G | F | G | G | G | G | G | G | G | G | F |
| Representativeness of sample (size, composition) | P | G | F | P | F | G | F | F | F | F | G | F | F | F | F | G | F |
| Is the study design appropriate for the research question? | F | F | F | P | G | G | F | P | P | F | G | F | F | F | F | G | P |
| **Overall Confidence Score** | L | M | M/L | L | M | H/M | M/L | L | L | M/L | H | L | L | M/L | M/L | H | L |

# SUMMARY AND DISCUSSION

## CONCLUSIONS AND RECOMMENDATIONS

In this section, we will summarize the results as they relate to the key questions and provide a series of recommendations for future research on rural health issues.

As evidenced by our review, there were several conditions for which there was a paucity of evidence regarding their prevention, diagnosis or treatment in rural health care settings (e.g., sexually transmitted diseases, rheumatoid arthritis, COPD, chronic pain, hepatitis C, anxiety disorders, substance use disorders, post-treatment cancer surveillance, traumatic brain injury). Studies tended to be conducted in areas in which either the information was readily available in a national database, a performance measure or guideline existed for which there was evidence and which served to operationalize quality care (e.g., via claims data), or a local health care problem existed that the authors were seeking to quantify. Given the data sources, study designs were predominantly cross-sectional or retrospective cohort designs, and only one of the studies we reviewed used a prospective design. Few studies associated health care differences with health outcomes. Given these limitations, the strength of the evidence was at best weak to moderate for most areas even when a significant finding was consistently present. This complicated interpretability. Most of our conclusions, therefore, are at best suggestive.

Another significant conceptual problem with the use of extant data sources and the cross-sectional study designs used was that potential reasons for rural-urban differences were often treated as confounders and adjusted for in statistical models. There are many correlates of rural residency that may affect health care utilization or access (e.g., lower rates of college graduates, types of health insurance, higher rates of poverty in highly rural areas, etc.).[119] Statistically adjusting for these contextual characteristics only to then find no difference between rural and urban residents in health outcomes does not mean that rural residents or, in some cases, urban residents are not disadvantaged.[120] Similar points have been made in discussions of race disparities,[121] with recommendations made to "unpack" the factors underlying the differences, which we feel are also applicable in this area.

Because our evidence base relied on peer reviewed articles, we did not include national reports examining potential differences in rural vs. urban health care. However, because these reports serve to inform policy makers, at the end of this section we compare findings from the 2010 National Healthcare Disparities Report[122] and the 2010 VHA Facility Quality and Safety Report[123] with the results of this systematic review.

## SUMMARY OF EVIDENCE BY KEY QUESTION

**Key Question #1. Do adults with health care needs who live in rural areas have different intermediate (e.g., HbA1c, Blood pressure, etc.) or final health care outcomes (i.e., mortality, morbidity, QOL) than those living in urban areas?**

Most of the evidence regarding potential differences in health care outcomes between rural and urban patients is weak either by the quality of the study designs and/or the paucity of studies evaluating whether any differences exist. Below we list the findings for which there is some evidence of a health care disparity.

- There is some weak evidence that increasing rurality is associated with a greater frequency of hospitalization for ACSC's.

- No evidence for differences in cancer mortality.

- There is some evidence of greater rates of DCIS and lower rates of invasive cervical cancer in urban areas where screening rates are higher.

- There was no evidence for a disparity between rural and urban patients with diabetes in terms of diabetes complications or the prevalence of ESRD. However, there was some evidence that race by rurality interactions may exist in diabetes care and in the treatment of ESRD.

- Although very limited, the available information suggests that outpatient control of hypertension, at least among veterans, does not differ between those residing in rural vs. urban areas.

There was weak evidence for higher hospitalization rates for rural residents treated for depression in Arkansas.

## Key Question #2. Is the structure (e.g., types of available providers) or the process (e.g., likelihood of referral) of health care different for adults with health care needs who live in urban vs. rural environments?

### Use of Medication

No consistent differences were found in receipt of or adherence to medication. To the extent that a few studies reported any differences, urban residents tended to receive more medications.

### Medical Procedures and Diagnostic Tests

The use of most services, including office visits and consultations, imaging services, and diagnostic testing, were found to be lower in rural areas compared to urban areas. More consistent evidence was found specifically for lower screening rates for breast and cervical cancer in many rural areas. Differences in screening rates for colorectal cancer are not consistently found. However, all but one study found a greater frequency of unstaged cancer at the time of diagnosis in rural areas compared to urban areas.

### Medical Appointments with Providers

Rural residents were less likely to see a medical provider than urban residents. Specifically, rural residents were less likely to see specialists, and low availability of specialists had deleterious impact on some health outcomes (e.g., cancer mortality). However, studies did not generally account for the fact that rural residents often receive specialty health care in urban clinics and how this might affect health outcomes. More consistent was the lower rate of mental health care service receipt among residents in rural areas.

*Usual Source of Care*

There was no consistent evidence that rural residents were less likely to have a usual source of care. In fact, there was more consistent evidence that rural residents had better continuity of care. Having fewer health care choices seems to increase the odds of remaining with the same provider over time.

*Provider Availability and Expertise*

There was consistent evidence that highly rural areas had a paucity of health care providers. There was some evidence that providers in some highly rural areas were more likely to be physician extenders (e.g., physician assistants, nurse practitioners). There was some weak evidence that physician extenders in some rural areas may not have comparable credentials to their urban counterparts. More consistent evidence was found indicating that rural residents were more likely to have primary care providers whose training was in family medicine rather than general internal medicine or OB/GYN. There was also consistent evidence that rural residents had less access to specialty medical services unless they traveled to urban health care centers. Fewer non-physician rehabilitation specialists are available in rural areas.

There was weak evidence provided by one study that suggested that limitations in provider knowledge might impact clinical practice viz. colorectal cancer screening.

The two studies examining the availability of rehabilitation specialists both found a paucity of such providers in many rural areas relative to urban areas. One of the studies compared availability over several years, increasing confidence in this finding. Similarly, there is a fairly consistent finding of fewer mental health specialists in rural areas.

*Quality of Care*

There were also no consistent differences between rural and urban areas in treatment quality measures for diabetes, although one study found evidence for regional variation in rural disparities. This was not assessed in other studies. Similarly, the two larger studies of treatment of hypertension did not find any quality differences between rural and urban settings.

Although the studies are few, there is some evidence suggesting that care for some conditions (e.g., HIV/AIDS) may be lower in rural areas. Two of three studies examining quality of cancer treatment indicated lower quality of care in rural areas. The third, however, found that rurality was less of a contributor to quality care differences than was provider characteristics.

**Key Question #3.   If there are differences in the structure or the process of health care in rural vs. urban environments, do those differences contribute to variation in overall or intermediate health outcomes for adults with health care needs?**

Although there were many studies that documented differences in health care structure or process between urban and rural health care settings, as we noted above few associated those differences with variation in health outcomes. The list of findings below is generally based on single studies of variable quality. Results can only be considered suggestive.

- Lower rates of mammography and cervical cancer screening in rural areas was associated with lower rates of ductal carcinoma *in situ* (vs. more invasive breast cancer) and higher rates of invasive cervical cancer in rural areas.

- Improving access by the creation of Rural Health Clinics in underserved areas was associated with improved adherence to treatment guidelines for diabetes.[52]

- Limited numbers of providers in rural areas may foster better continuity of care.

- Limitations in provider availability may be associated with increased odds of hospitalization among older rural residents for ACSCs.

Two studies that were published after our sampling frame demonstrate comparable rates of pharmacotherapy for rural and urban residents with depression and rural vs. urban veterans with depression or anxiety disorders.[124,125] Both studies found that the odds of having psychotherapy appointments, however, were lower among those who lived in rural settings, and that this difference was mediated by provider availability.

## Key Question #4.  If there are differences in intermediate or final health outcomes for adult patients with health care needs, what systems factors other than those due to differences in health care structure or process moderate those differences (e.g., travel distance)?

*Insurance*

- Lack of insurance was associated with increased odds of ACSC associated admissions, but this was not limited to rural residents; however, within rural areas those who had supplemental HMO plans had fewer admissions compared to older residence with a fee-for-service insurance plan. Of note, one study found that Medicare HMO enrollees had to travel further for acute care services than Medicare fee-for-service patients, and were less likely to receive services within their county.[126]

*Travel Distance*

- There was limited evidence that having a greater distance to treatment decreased odds of receipt of radiotherapy for older women with breast cancer, aftercare for veterans treated in inpatient alcohol treatment programs, and frequency of mental health appointments.

- The presence of Rural Health Clinics in underserved areas improved treatment access and adherence to treatment guidelines for patients with diabetes.

*Patient Attitude*

- There is some weak evidence that urban residents may have a lower threshold for seeking mental health care than do rural residents, and that this may be related to differential use of mental health services.

*Race Disparities*

- For many conditions covered in this review, race disparities were greater in urban than in rural areas. This was observed in admissions for ACSC-related conditions, stage at presentation for colorectal and prostate cancers, detection of diabetes, secondary prevention for diabetes-related conditions, post-hospitalization continuity of care for mental illness, and, among Native Americans, the odds of receiving a kidney transplant.

- Race disparities were greater in rural areas for mortality rates among Hispanics for ESRD and for rates of organ transplants for blacks.

The 2010 National Healthcare Disparities Report (NHDR) compared health outcomes between noncore areas (defined as rural counties without metropolitan or micropolitan areas) with large fringe metropolitan areas (defined as suburban counties of metropolitan areas with one million or more residents).[122] Most of their findings relating to adult ambulatory healthcare, found results comparable to this review. Specifically, the NHDR also found evidence for increased hospitalizations for ACSC's, elevated suicide rates, reduced rates of CRC screens and lower insurance rates among rural residents. Differences in the NHDR and this review were only noted for lung and CRC related mortality rates and the odds of flu vaccination (they found disparities, we found the evidence to be inconsistent for cancer care). Importantly, it must be noted that the studies covered by this review most often compared rural areas with *urban* areas, not suburban areas. Given that we found urban disparities in some healthcare areas (notably cancer care), this might account for the differential findings. Finally, the NHDR reported differences in a few areas for which no articles were included in this review -- advice for exercise among obese patients and the five year odds of cholesterol screening -- both of which demonstrated a rural disadvantage.

The 2010 VHA Facility Quality and Safety Report compared US census defined urban areas with non-urban areas (called rural, but which would include suburban counties).[123] Only bivariate findings are included in the report. Comparable to this evidence synthesis, no differences were noted for guideline concordant follow-up care for patients with diabetes, control of hypertension, or immunization rates for influenza. Also assessed in that report, but not covered by this evidence synthesis, were patient satisfaction, counseling for tobacco cessation and mental health screens, none of which demonstrated consistent differences between rural and urban areas nationally. Despite the similarities, it is difficult to conclude that no differences between highly rural and urban (or suburban) areas exist because of the way VA categorizes urban vs. rural.

## RESEARCH IMPLICATIONS AND RECOMMENDATIONS

As has been shown by others, the definition of rural that is used in a study has a significant impact on the findings and, consequently, the policy implications.[11,12,14] Yet, there is little consistency across studies either in terms of what convention is used to define rural or how a chosen convention is actually employed in the study. Consequently, we make the following recommendations for researchers regarding definitions of "rural" and other methodologic issues based on our observations and the work of others.[11,12,14]

1. Specify the convention that was used to define "rural" in the study and how it was specifically operationalized. Many studies use rural–urban commuting area codes (RUCA) as their starting point, but then combine the categories in unique ways. The convention used by VA may minimize rural-urban disparities for some healthcare services. A more graded convention (e.g., RUCA, RUCC or UIC) would allow for better identification of areas in need of intervention.

2.  Provide a rationale for why the convention used in the study was chosen and the potential impact of that choice on the research question (e.g., Is a monotonic relationship between levels of population density and the outcome variable expected?).

    a.  Consider using a statistical method for deciding between conventions if more than one option is available.[12]

3.  If the study questions do not call for a clear choice in the convention to be used, consider using more than one convention and reporting the results for both definitions.

4.  Provide a rationale for the unit of analysis viz. the research question. For example, does the unit of analysis reflect the functioning of local health care systems or markets (e.g., county vs. zip code as unit of analysis) or is the focus individual health outcomes?

    a.  Associations between health care parameters and specific health outcomes found when using aggregate units (e.g., counties or zip codes) may not hold at the individual level (i.e., a modifiable areal unit problem). This limitation was generally not acknowledged.

As noted by Rost et al.,[127] many of the important questions concerning rural-urban disparities in health care cannot be answered by simply demonstrating differences in health care systems. A more useful set of questions focus on clarifying what health outcomes, if any, show a disparity, for whom does the disparity exist, and why is there a disparity. Accordingly, we make the following recommendations.

1.  Because many factors are correlated with rurality, adjusting for all available covariates may lead to false conclusions regarding the association of rurality and study outcomes, and provide insufficient information for the development of healthcare policy. For most research questions, a more contextual analytic approach should be used.

    a.  For example, first reporting bivariate associations (missing from many papers) and then examining which, if any, of the available covariates significant in multivariable models contributed to the observed differences in the bivariate analyses. Alternatively, other statistical models, such as multilevel models, might be useful.

    b.  These associations must also be considered when selecting instrumental variables or developing propensity models for risk adjustment.

2.  Most rural residents receive their primary health care locally. However, a significant proportion of rural residents will travel to more urban areas for medical conditions that require specialist treatment or for which they have less confidence in the expertise of their usual provider[111] Few studies acknowledged this trend, and those that did generally omitted data from those individuals who received their care in urban settings. Studies should address this selection bias and seek to understand its implications for their study findings and for the health care systems involved.

3.  In several studies, interactions were found between race (and/or income) and residential population density. Such interactions may have significant implications for interventions designed to address a rural health disparity, and should be tested in the research model if

appropriate. Interactions between race and rurality should be further explored as they could reflect any of the following (see Stern, 2010[12] for a discussion):

a. Living in a rural or urban area affects health care (or access to health care) for a minority group differently than it does for whites.

b. The association is due to the distribution of minority members of the patient group in question.

c. A third factor is associated with both race and rurality (e.g., poverty)

d. There is an association between race and some aspect of the healthcare system (e.g., proportion of providers who are minorities).

4. Studies that describe differences in healthcare systems but do not associate such differences with health outcomes are of limited value. Areas with limited healthcare resources may engage in successful service substitution and areas with an abundance of health care resources may engage in overutilization.

5. Only one of the studies we reviewed that compared rural with urban health care used a prospective design. This limits the confidence with which factors associated with a rural disparity can be considered as potentially causal.

6. Studies focused on providing descriptions of barriers to care are only helpful insofar as the barriers are associated with actual limitations in the use of needed healthcare services. All consumers have barriers to care, but not all barriers limit health care seeking.

7. Large national databases often involve statistical corrections to adjust for any potential sampling bias. Using such databases improves a study's external validity; however, the findings from such secondary analyses are often limited by what measures are available in the database.

8. Studies that relied on self-report measures rarely assessed or corrected for sampling bias, and many did not include sampling bias as a possible study limitation. Similarly, studies sampling from multiple sites often did not address potential clustering effects in their analyses.

9. Studies that sample nationally should consider examining whether there is regional variation in observed rural-urban disparities. Regional variation in rural-urban disparities has been demonstrated in studies involving veterans[4] and non-veterans.[31,51] Pooling across regions may attenuate disparities. Moreover, health care systems operate locally and identifying areas where problems are greatest would help policy makers target areas that have the most need.

There are large gaps in the evidence base across clinical conditions, and minimal empirical work conducted on several areas of particular interest to the VA (e.g., TBI, PTSD, Hepatitis C). Filling in the evidence base will allow VA policy planners to make informed decisions about resource allocation.

# REFERENCES

1.     Veterans Health Administration, Department of Veterans Affairs, Office of Rural Health. About Rural Veterans. Available at: http://vaww.ruralhealth.va.gov/RURALHEALTH/ About_Rural_Veterans.asp. Accessed April 29, 2011.

2.     United States Department of Agriculture. Rural Population and Migration, 2009. Available at: http://www.ers.usda.gov/Briefing/Population/. Accessed April 29, 2011.

3.     Veterans Health Administration, Department of Veterans Affairs, Office of Rural Health. Demographic Characteristics of Rural Veterans. Available at: http://vaww.ruralhealth. va.gov/RURALHEALTH/docs/IBDemographicCharacteristics.pdf. Accessed April 29, 2011.

4.     Weeks WB, Kazis LE, Shen Y. Differences in health-related quality of life in rural and urban veterans. *Am J Public Health* 2004;94(10):1762-7.

5.     Weeks WB, Wallace AE, Wang S, Lee A, Kazis LE. Rural-urban disparities in health-related quality of life within disease categories of Veterans. *J Rural Health* 2006;22(3):204-11.

6.     Wallace AE, MacKenzie TA, Wright SM, Weeks WB. A cross-sectional, multi-year examination of rural and urban Veterans Administration users: 2002-2006. *Mil Med* 2010;175(4):252-8.

7.     Wallace AE, Lee R, MacKenzie TA, et al. A longitudinal analysis of rural and urban veterans' health-related quality of life. *J Rural Health* 2010;26(2):156-63.

8.     Weeks WB, Bott DM, Lamkin PR, Wright SM. Veterans Health Administration and Medicare outpatient health care utilization by older rural and urban New England veterans. *J Rural Health* 2005;21(2):167-71.

9.     West AN, Weeks WB. Health care expenditures for urban and rural veterans in veterans health administration care. *Health Serv Res* 2009;44(5 Pt 1):1718-34.

10.    Institute of Medicine. Unequal treatment: confronting racial and ethnic disparities in health care. Washington DC: The National Academies Press, 2003.

11.    Weeks WB, Wallace AE, West AN, Heady HR, Hawthorne K. Research on rural veterans: An analysis of the literature. *J Rural Health* 2008;24(4):337-44.

12.    Stern S, Merwin E, Hauenstein E, et al. The effects of rurality on mental and physical health. *Health Serv Outcomes Res Methods* 2010;10:33-66.

13.    West AN, Lee RE, Shambaugh-Miller ME, et al. Defining "rural" for veterans' health care planning. *J Rural Health* 2010;26(4):301-9.

14.    Berke EM, West AN, Wallace AE, Weeks WB. Practical and policy implications of using different rural-urban classification systems: a case study of inpatient service utilization among Veterans Administration users. *J Rural Health* 2009;25(3):259-66.

15.   Institute of Medicine. Redesigning the clinical effectiveness research paradigm: Innovation and practice-based approaches: Workshop summary. Olsen L, McGinnis JM, eds. Washington DC: The National Academies Press, 2010.

16.   Owens DK, Lohr KN, Atkins D, et al. Grading the strength of a body of evidence when comparing medical interventions-Agency for Healthcare Research and Quality and the Effective Health Care Program. *J Clin Epidemiol* 2009;63:513-23.

17.   Shamliyan TA, Kane RL, Ansari M, et al. Development quality criteria to evaluate nontherapeutic studies of incidence, prevalence, or risk factors of chronic diseases: pilot study of new checklists. *J Clin Epidemiol* 2011;64:637-57.

18.   Casey MM, Thiede Call K, Klinger JM. Are rural residents less likely to obtain recommended preventive healthcare services? *Am J Prev Med* 2001;21:182-8.

19.   Zhang P, Tao G, Irwin KL. Utilization of preventive medical services in the United States: a comparison between rural and urban populations. *J Rural Health* 2000;16(4):349-56.

20.   Brown KC, Fitzhugh EC, Neutens JJ, Klein DA. Screening mammography utilization in Tennessee women: The association with residence. *J Rural Health* 2009;25:167-73.

21.   Coughlin SS, Leadbetter S, Richards T, Sabatino SA. Contextual analysis of breast and cervical cancer screening and factors associated with health care access among United States women, 2002. *Soc Sci Med* 2008;66:260-75.

22.   Coughlin SS, Thompson TD. Colorectal cancer screening practices among men and women in rural and nonrural areas of the United States, 1999. *J Rural Health* 2004;20:118-24.

23.   Coughlin SS, Thompson TD, Hall HI, Logan P, Uhler RJ. Breast and cervical carcinoma screening practices among women in rural and nonrural areas of the United States, 1998-1999. *Cancer* 2002;94:2801-12.

24.   Kinney AY, Harrell J, Slattery M, Martin C, Sandler RS. Rural-urban differences in colon cancer risk in blacks and whites: the North Carolina Colon Cancer Study. *J Rural Health* 2006;22(2):124-30.

25.   Schootman M, Fuortes LJ. Breast and cervical carcinoma: The correlation of activity limitations and rurality with screening, disease incidence, and mortality. *Cancer* 1999a;86(6):1087-94.

26.   Stearns SC, Slifkin, RT, Edin HM. Access to care for rural Medicare beneficiaries. *J Rural Health* 2000;16(1):31-42.

27.   Epstein B, Grant T, Schiff M, Kasehagen L. Does rural residence affect access to prenatal care in Oregon? *J Rural Health* 2009;25:150-157.

28.   Laditka JN, Laditka SB, Probst JC. Health care access in rural areas: Evidence that hospitalization for ambulatory care-sensitive conditions in the United States may increase with the level of rurality. *Health Place* 2009;15(3):761-70.

29.    Saag KG, Doebbeling BN, Rohrer JE, et al. Variation in tertiary prevention and health service utilization among the elderly: The role of urban-rural residence and supplemental insurance. *Med Care* 1998;36:965-76.

30.    Schreiber S, Zielinski T. The meaning of ambulatory care sensitive admissions: urban and rural perspectives. *J Rural Health* 1997;13(4):276-84.

31.    Edwards JB, Tudiver F. Women's preventive screening in Rural Health Clinics. *Women's Health Issues* 2008;18(3):155-66.

32.    Probst JC, Laditka JN, Laditka SB. Association between community health center and rural health clinic presence and county-level hospitalization rates for ambulatory care sensitive conditions: an analysis across eight US states. *BMC Health Serv Res* 2009;9:134. Epub 2009 31 July.

33.    Shugarman LR, Sorbero ME, Tian H, Jain AK, Ashwood JS. An exploration of urban and rural differences in lung cancer survival among Medicare beneficiaries. *Am J Public Health* 2008;98(7):1280-7.

34.    Loberiza FR, Cannon AJ, Weisenburger DD, et al. Survival disparities in patients with lymphoma according to place of residence and treatment provider: A population based study. *J Clin Oncol* 2009;27:5376-82.

35.    Elliott TE, Elliott BA, Renier CM, Haller IV. Rural-urban differences in cancer care: results from the Lake Superior Rural Cancer Care Project. *Minn Med* 2004;87(9):44-50.

36.    Chirumbole M, Gusani N, Howard A, Leonard T, Lewis P, Muscat J. A comparison of stage of presentation for pancreatic and colorectal cancer in Pennsylvania 2000-2005. *Anticancer Res* 2009;29:3427-32.

37.    Higginbotham JC, Moulder J, Currier M. Rural v. urban aspects of cancer: first-year data from the Mississippi Central Cancer Registry. *Fam Community Health* 2001;24(2):1-9.

38.    Paquette I, Finlayson SRG. Rural versus urban colorectal and lung cancer patients: Differences in stage at presentation. *J Am Coll Surg* 2007;205(5):636-41.

39.    McLafferty S, Wang F. Rural reversal? Rural-urban disparities in late-stage cancer risk in Illinois. *Cancer* 2009;115:2755-64.

40.    Sankaranarayanan J, Watanabe-Galloway S, Sun J, Qiu F, Boilesen E, Thorson AG. Rurality and other determinants of early colorectal cancer diagnosis in Nebraska: A 6-year cancer registry study, 1998-2003. *J Rural Health* 2009;25:358-65.

41.    McLaughlin J, Balkrishnan R, Paskett ED, Kimmick GG, Anderson RT. Patient and provider determinants associated with the prescription of adjuvant hormonal therapies following a diagnosis of breast cancer in Medicaid-enrolled patients. *J Natl Med Assoc* 2009;101:1112-8.

42.    Schootman M, Aft R. Rural-urban differences in radiation therapy for ductal carcinoma in-situ of the breast. *Breast Cancer Res Treat* 2001;68(2):117-25.

43.    Baldwin LM, Cai Y, Larson EH, et al. Access to cancer services for rural colorectal cancer patients. *J Rural Health* 2008;24(4):390-9.

44.    O'Hare AM, Johansen KL, Rodriguez RA. Dialysis and kidney transplantation among patients living in rural areas of the United States. *Kidney Int* 2006;69(2):343-9.

45.    Krishna S, Gillespie KN, McBride TM. Diabetes burden and access to preventive care in the rural United States. *J Rural Health* 2010;26(1):3-11.

46.    Ward MM. Access to care and the incidence of end-stage renal disease due to diabetes. *Diabetes Care* 2009;32(6):1032-6.

47.    Andrus MR, Kelley KW, Murphey LM, Herndon KC. A comparison of diabetes care in rural and urban medical clinics in Alabama. *J Community Health* 2004;29(1):29-44.

48.    Koopman RJ, Mainous AG, Geesey ME. Rural residence and Hispanic ethnicity: Doubly disadvantaged for diabetes? *J Rural Health* 2006;25:63-8.

49.    Morden NE, Berke EM, Welsh DE, McCarthy JF, MacKenzie TA, Kilbourne AM. Quality of care for cardiometabolic disease: Associations with mental disorder and rurality. *Med Care* 2010;48:72-78.

50.    Rosenblatt RA, Baldwin L-M, Chan L, et al. Improving the quality of outpatient care for older patients with diabetes: lessons from a comparison of rural and urban communities. *J Fam Pract* 2001;50(8):676-80.

51.    Weingarten JP, Brittman S, Hu W, Przybyszewski C, Hammond JM, FitzGerald D. The state of diabetes care provided to Medicare beneficiaries living in rural America. *J Rural Health* 2006;22(4):351-8.

52.    Kirkbride K, Wallace N. Rural health clinics and diabetes-related primary care for Medicaid beneficiaries in Oregon. *J Rural Health* 2009;25:247-52.

53.    Hicks PC Bublitz Emsermann C, Westfall JM, Parnes B. Comparison of HTN management in patients with diabetes between rural and urban primary care clinics in Northeastern Colorado – a report from SNOCAP. *Rural Remote Health* 2010;10:1279. Epub 2010 Feb 12.

54.    King DE, Crisp JR. Rural-urban differences in factors associated with poor blood pressure control among outpatients. *South Med J* 2006;99(11):1221-3.

55.    Colleran KM, Richards A, Shafer K. Disparities in cardiovascular disease risk and treatment: demographic comparison. *J Investig Med* 2007;55(8):415-22.

56.    Dellasega C, Orwig D, Ahern F, Lenz E. Postdischarge medication use of elderly cardiac patients from urban and rural locations. *J Gerontol A Biol Sci Med Sci* 1999;54A:M514-20.

57.    Whyte BM, Carr JC. Comparison of AIDS in women in rural and urban Georgia. *South Med J* 1992;85(6):571-8.

58.  Cohn SE, Berk ML, Berry SH, et al. The care of HIV-infected adults in rural areas of the United States. *J Acquir Immune Defic Syndr* 2001;28(4):385-92.

59.  Napravnik S, Eron JJ, McKaig RG, Hein AD, Menezes P, Quinlivan EB. Factors associated with fewer visits for HIV primary care at a tertiary care center in the Southeastern U.S. *AIDS Care* 2006;18(Suppl 1):S45-50.

60.  Schur CL, Berk ML, Dunbar JR, Shapiro MF, Cohn SE, Bozzette SA. Where to seek care: An examination of people in rural areas with HIV/AIDS. *J Rural Health* 2002;18;337-47.

61.  Buchanan RJ, Schiffer R, Stuifbergen A, et al. Demographic and disease characteristics of people with multiple sclerosis living in urban and rural areas. *Int J MS Care* 2006a;8(3):89-98.

62.  Buchanan RJ, Wang S, Stuifbergen A, Chakravorty BJ, Zhu L, Kim M. Urban/rural differences in the use of physician services by people with multiple sclerosis. *NeuroRehabilitation* 2006b;21(3):177-87.

63.  Buchanan RJ, Schiffer R, Wang S, et al. Satisfaction with mental health care among people with multiple sclerosis in urban and rural areas. *Psychiatr Serv* 2006c;57(8):1206-9.

64.  Schootman M, Fuortes L. Functional status following traumatic brain injuries: population-based rural-urban differences. *Brain Inj* 1999b;13:995-1004.

65.  Johnstone B, Nossaman LD, Schopp LH, Holmquist L, Rupright SJ. Distribution of services and supports for people with traumatic brain injury in rural and urban Missouri. *J Rural Health* 2002;18:109-17.

66.  Wilson RD, Lewis SA, Murray PK. Trends in the rehabilitation therapist workforce in underserved areas: 1980-2000. *J Rural Health* 2009;25:26-32.

67.  Gibbons RD, Hur K, Bhaumik DK, Mann JJ. The relationship between antidepressant medication use and rate of suicide. *Arch Gen Psychiatry* 2005;62(2):165-72.

68.  Fiske A, Gatz M, Hannell E. Rural suicide rates and availability of health care providers. *J Community Psychol* 2005;33(5):537-43.

69.  Rost K, Zhang M, Fortney J, Smith J, Smith GR. Rural-urban differences in depression treatment and suicidality. *Med Care* 1998;36(7):1098-107.

70.  Fortney J, Rushton G, Wood S, et al. Community-level risk factors for depression hospitalizations. *Adm Policy Ment Health & Ment Health Serv Res* 2007;34:343-52.

71.  Fortney JC, Xu S, Dong F. Community-level correlates of hospitalizations for persons with schizophrenia. *Psychiatr Serv* 2009 60:772-8.

72.  Farrell SP, Koch JR, Blank M. Rural and urban differences in continuity of care after state hospital discharge. *Psychiatr Serv* 1996;47(6):652-4.

73.    Fischer EP, McSweeney JC, Pyne JM, et al. Influence of family involvement and substance use on sustained utilization of services for schizophrenia. *Psychiatr Serv* 2008;59(8):902-8.

74.    Fortney J, Rost K, Zhang M, Warren J. The impact of geographic accessibility on the intensity and quality of depression treatment. *Med Care* 1999;37:884-93.

75.    Mohamed S, Neale M, Rosenheck RA. VA intensive mental health case management in urban and rural areas: veteran characteristics and service delivery. *Psychiatr Serv* 2009;60(7):914-21.

76.    Rost K, Owen RR, Smith J, Smith GR. Rural-urban differences in service use and course of illness in bipolar disorder. *J Rural Health* 1998;14(1):36-43.

77.    Rost K, Fortney J, Zhang M, Smith J, Smith GR. Treatment of depression in rural Arkansas: policy implications for improving care. *J Rural Health* 1999;15(3):308-15.

78.    Rost K, Adams S, Xu S, Dong F. Rural-urban differences in hospitalization rates of primary care patients with depression. *Psychiatr Serv* 2007;58(4):503-8.

79.    Elhai JD, Baugher SN, Quevillon RP, Sauvageot J, Frueh BC. Psychiatric symptoms and health service utilization in rural and urban combat veterans with posttraumatic stress disorder. *J Nerv Ment Dis* 2004;192(10):701-4.

80.    Booth BM, Kirchner J, Fortney J, Ross R, Rost K. Rural at-risk drinkers: correlates and one-year use of alcoholism treatment services. *J Stud Alcohol* 2000;61(2):267-77.

81.    Grant BF. Toward an alcohol treatment model: a comparison of treated and untreated respondents with DSM-IV alcohol use disorders in the general population. *Alcohol Clin Exp Res* 1996;20(2):372-8.

82.    Metsch LR, McCoy CB. Drug treatment experiences: rural and urban comparisons. *Subst Use Misuse* 1999;34(4-5):763-84.

83.    Robertson EB, Donnermeyer JF. Illegal drug use among rural adults: mental health consequences and treatment utilization. *Am J Drug Alcohol Abuse* 1997;23(3):467-84.

84.    Fortney JC, Booth BM, Blow FC, Bunn JY, Loveland Cook CA. The effects of travel barriers and age on the utilization of alcoholism treatment aftercare. *Am J Drug Alcohol Abuse* 1995;21(3):391-406.

85.    Petterson SM. Metropolitan-nonmetropolitan differences in amount and type of mental health treatment. *Arch Psychiatr Nurs* 2003;17(1):12-9.

86.    Petterson S, Williams IC, Hauenstein EJ, Rovnyak V, Merwin E. Race and ethnicity and rural mental health treatment. *J Health Care Poor Underserved* 2009;20(3):662-77.

87.    Hauenstein EJ, Petterson S, Merwin E, Rovnyak V, Heise B, Wagner D. Rurality, gender, and mental health treatment. *Fam Community Health* 2006;29(3):169-85.

88.   Wang PS, Lane, M, Olfson M, Pincus, HA, Wells KB, Kessler RC. Twelve-month use of mental health services in the United States: Results from the National Comorbidity Survey Replication. *Arch Gen Psychiatry* 2005;62(6):629-40.

89.   Fillenbaum GG, Hanlon JT, Corder EH, Ziqubu-Page T, Wall WE, Brock D. Prescription and nonprescription drug use among black and white community-residing elderly. *Am J Public Health* 1993;83(11):1577-82.

90.   Hanlon JT, Landerman LR, Wall WE, et al. Is medication use by community-dwelling elderly people influenced by cognitive function? *Age Aging* 1996;25(3):190-6.

91.   Lago D, Stuart B, Ahern F. Rurality and prescription drug utilization among the elderly: an archival study. *J Rural Health* 1993;9(1):6-16.

92.   Lillard LA, Rogowski J, Kington R. Insurance coverage for prescription drugs: effects on use and expenditures in the Medicare population. *Med Care* 1999;37(9):926-36.

93.   Mueller C, Schur C. Insurance coverage of prescription drugs and the rural elderly. *J Rural Health* 2004;20(1):17-25.

94.   Xu KT, Smith SR, Borders TF. Access to prescription drugs among noninstitutionalized elderly people in west Texas. *Am J Health-Syst Pharm* 2003;60:675-82.

95.   Rogowski J, Lillard LA, Kington R. The financial burden of prescription drug use among elderly persons. *Gerontologist* 1997;37(4):475-82.

96.   Miller ME, Holahan J, Welch WP. Geographic variations in physician service utilization. *Med Care Res Rev* 1995;52(2):252-78.

97.   Escarce JJ, Epstein KR, Colby DC, Schwartz JS. Racial differences in the elderly's use of medical procedures and diagnostic tests. *Am J Public Health* 1993;83(7):948-54.

98.   Blazer DG, Landerman LR, Fillenbaum G, Horner R. Health services access and use among older adults in North Carolina: urban vs rural residents. *Am J Public Health* 1995;85(10):1384-90.

99.   McConnel CE, Zetzman MR. Urban/rural differences in health service utilization by elderly persons in the United States. *J Rural Health* 1993;9(4):270-80.

100.  Glover S, Moore CG, Probs JC, Samuels ME. Disparities in access to care among rural working-age adults. *J Rural Health* 2004;20(3):193-205.

101.  Himes CL, Rutrough TS. Differences in the use of health services by metropolitan and nonmetropolitan elderly. *J Rural Health* 1994;10(2):80-8.

102.  Larson SL, Fleishman JA. Rural-urban differences in usual source of care and ambulatory service use: analyses of national data using Urban Influence Codes. *Med Care* 2003;41(7 Suppl):III-65-74.

103.  Mueller KJ, Patil K, Boilesen E. The role of uninsurance and race in healthcare utilization by rural minorities. *Health Serv Res* 1998;33(3 Pt 1):597-610.

104.  Maciejewski ML, Perkins M, Li Y-F, Chapko M, Fortney JC, Liu C-F. Utilization and expenditures of veterans obtaining primary care in community clinis and VA medical centers: an observational cohort study. *BMC Health Serv Res* 2007;7:56. Epub 2007 18 April.

105.  Fortney JC, Borowsky SJ, Hedeen AN, Maciejewski ML, Chapko MK. VA Community-Based Outpatient Clinics: Access and utilization performance measures. *Med Care* 2002;40(7):561-9.

106.  Meza JL, Chen L-W, William TV, Ullrich F, Mueller KJ. Differences in beneficiary assessments of health care between TRICARE Prime and TRICARE Prime Remote. *Mil Med* 2006;171(10):950-4.

107.  Borders TF. Rural community-dwelling elders' reports of access to care: are there Hispanic versus non-Hispanic white disparities? *J Rural Health* 2004;20(3):210-20.

108.  Rohrer JE, Kruse G, Zhang Y. Hispanic ethnicity, rural residence, and regular source of care. *J Community Health* 2004;29(1):1-13.

109.  Brown B, Bushardt R, Harmon K, Nguyen SA. Dermatology diagnoses among rural and urban physician assistants. *JAAPA* 2009;22(12):32-5.

110.  Ferrer RL. Pursuing equity: Contact with primary care and specialist clinicians by demographics, insurance, and health status. *Ann Fam Med* 2007;5(6):492-502.

111.  Biola H, Pathman DE. Are there enough doctors in my rural community? Perceptions of the local physician supply. *J Rural Health* 2009;25(2):115-23.

112.  Grumbach K, Hart LG, Mertz E, Coffman J, Palazzo L. Who is caring for the underserved? A comparison of primary care physicians and nonphysician clinicians in California and Washington. *Ann Fam Med* 2003;1(2):97-104.

113.  Everett CM, Schumacher JR, Wright A, Smith MA. Physician assistants and nurse practitioners as a usual source of care. *J Rural Health* 2009;25(4):407-14.

114.  Jones PE. Doctor and physician assistant distribution in rural and remote Texas counties. *Aust J Rural Health* 2008;16(6):389.

115.  Gunderson A, Menachemi N, Brummel-Smith K, Brooks R. Physicians who treat the elderly in rural Florida: trends indicating concerns regarding access to care. *J Rural Health* 2006;2(3):224-8.

116.  Menachemi N, Brooks RG, Clawson A, Stine C, Beitsch L. Continuing decline in service delivery for family physicians: is the malpractice crisis playing a role? *Qual Manag Health Care* 2006;15(1):39-45.

117.  Baldwin LM, Rosenblatt RA, Schneeweiss R, Lishner DM, Hart LG. Rural and urban physicians: does the content of their Medicare practices differ? *J Rural Health* 1999;15(2):240-251.

118.  Strickland WJ, Strickland DL, Garretson C. Rural and urban nonphysician providers in Georgia. *J Rural Health* 1998;14(2):109-20.

119.  United States Census Bureau. 2009 American Community Survey 1-Year Estimates, Geographic Comparison Tables, 2009. Available at: http://factfinder.census.gov/servlet/ DatasetMainPageServlet?_program=ACS. Accessed April 29, 2011.

120.  Brookhart MA, Stümer T, Glynn RJ, Rassen J, Schneeweiss S. Confounding control in healthcare database research: challenges and potential approaches. *Med Care* 2010;48(6 Suppl):S114-20.

121.  Walsh ME, Katz MA, Sechrest L. Unpacking cultural factors in adaptation to type 2 diabetes mellitus. *Med Care* 2002;40(1 Suppl):I129-39.

122.  United States Department of Health and Human Services, Agency for Healthcare Research and Quality. National Healthcare Disparities Report, 2010. Available at: http:// www.ahrq.gov/qual/qrdr10.htm. Accessed April 29, 2011.

123.  Veterans Health Administration, Department of Veterans Affairs. 2010 VHA Facility Quality and Safety Report, 2010. Available at: http://www.va.gov/health/docs/Hospital-ReportCard2010.pdf. Accessed April 29, 2011.

124.  Cully JA, Lameson JP, Phillips LL, Kunik ME, Fortney JC. Use of psychotherapy by rural and urban veterans. *J Rural Health* 2010;26:225-33.

125.  Fortney JC, Harman JS, Xu S, Dong F. The association between rural residence and the use, type, and quality of depression care. *J Rural Health* 2010;26:205-13.

126.  O'Neill L. The effect of insurance status on travel time for rural Medicare patients. *Med Care Res Rev* 2004;61(2):187-202.

127.  Rost K, Fortney J, Fischer E, Smith J. Use, quality, and outcomes of care for mental health: the rural perspective. *Med Care Res Rev* 2002;59(3):231-65.

Rural vs. Urban Ambulatory Health Care: A Systematic Review

Evidence-based Synthesis Program

# APPENDIX A.  DATA ABSTRACTION FORM

| Name of Study | | | | Check if Background paper ☐ |
|---|---|---|---|---|

| Journal | | First Author | Year | Inclusion Eligibility?  Y  N   If "No", what #? |
|---|---|---|---|---|

| Study Design | Cohort | Cross-sectional | Case-control | RCT | Non-RCT | Review/Meta-analysis |
|---|---|---|---|---|---|---|
| | | | | | | |

| Sample | Unit | # sites/ national? | Sample size | Vet?  Y  N | Rural/ urban?  Y  N | Rural definition used |
|---|---|---|---|---|---|---|

| Data Source | Registry | Survey (note response rate) | Health care Records | Primary vs. secondary  1°  2° | National database (define) | Date(s) of dataset |
|---|---|---|---|---|---|---|

| Analyses | Stat method | | Adjusted Covariates/Independent Variables | |
|---|---|---|---|---|
| | | | Appropriate Stats? | Y  N  N/A |
| | | | Adjusted for sampling bias? | Y  N  N/A |
| | | | Adjusted for non-response bias? | Y  N  N/A |
| | | | Adjusted for clustering? | Y  N  N/A |

**Findings:   Include outcome measures and, if appropriate, magnitude of effect.**

| Outcome Measure | 1 | 2 | 3 | 4 | 4a |
|---|---|---|---|---|---|
| Question | | | | | |

# APPENDIX B. PEER REVIEW COMMENTS AND AUTHOR RESPONSES

| REVIEWER COMMENT | RESPONSE |
|---|---|
| **1.  Are the objectives, scope, and methods for this review clearly described?** | |
| Yes. This is a good review. | Thank you. |
| Yes, although I think it will be important to highlight that this review is comparing the care of rural vs. urban patients in general, and that *data for rural vs. urban veterans are even more sparse and therefore one cannot infer that rural veterans face the same disparities in care as rural non-veterans.* | We agree, and have clarified this in the text. |
| Yes | |
| Yes. The objectives, scope, and methods make sense and are useful for researchers, providers, and policymakers. More work of this kind is needed. It is not clear why only ambulatory care articles were included in the study selection when some of the topics were relevant beyond only ambulatory care. The repeated mention of inconsistencies and other problems related to definitions of rurality and the way "rural vs. urban" is viewed conceptually were very important. More detailed suggestions about what needs to be done to address this (e.g., how will consensus be reached) would be helpful. More explicit information is needed about the study selection, data abstractions, data synthesis, and rating of the body of evidence. It would be hard to replicate this review with the information given. | We focused on ambulatory care. Including hospital care would have made the review unwieldy and too diffusely focused. That being said, some traditionally non-ambulatory care topics were included because they were indirect indicators of ambulatory care access and/or quality (e.g., hospitalizations for ambulatory care sensitive conditions). We have further clarified our methodology in the text. |
| a. Yes, though the methods could be expanded. It is difficult to assess the quality or thoroughness of the search for relevant articles, as the description of the process is minimal. Data abstractions were done by "researchers trained in critical analysis of the literature," but there is no description of the evaluation or of the qualifications of the abstractors. There is a bit more description of the evaluative ratings of the studies that were reviewed, but no mention of who did these ratings or of any inter-rater reliability.<br><br>b. Another concern is that the tables in which you present your ratings of the quality of the studies do not seem to be reflected in the text. For example, in a table, you give two studies low confidence ratings. But in the text, there is no indication that there may be problems with those studies. As one reads the text, the only way he would know that you have doubts about the quality of these studies would be to continually refer to the table at the end of the section. Few readers will do this. Within each section of text, you might want to segregate the good studies form the bad ones so the reader will know which ones to rely most on. | These are both excellent points and we have made relevant revisions in the text. |
| Yes | |
| Yes | |
| Yes | |
| **2.  Is there any indication of bias in our synthesis of the evidence?** | |
| No | |

Rural vs. Urban Ambulatory Health Care: A Systematic Review

Evidence-based Synthesis Program

| REVIEWER COMMENT | RESPONSE |
|---|---|
| No. This is a balanced and objective review that highlights the lack of good information and the inability to draw any firm conclusions. | Thank you. |
| No | |
| While there is no strong indication of bias, sources of bias could be better protected against through specific efforts. The methods used for review would be strengthened by blinding reviewers to both author and journal. Inter-rater reliability could be tested by more than one reviewer reviewing the same articles. It is unclear what preparation the reviewers had and how the reviewers were instructed and trained for this purpose. The term "trained reviewer" is used several times without much explanation about what that means. There is variation in that term. | We have elaborated on the methodology in the text to address the issues raised. The first and second authors rated all papers after jointly rating 20 to achieve consensus in our ratings. Since there is no evidence based rating system for non-randomized trials, we had to develop our own. In the text, we acknowledged that the ratings were qualitative in nature and that their primary value was to explicate to the readers the bases of our evaluations. |
| No – as you note, the evidence is pretty inconclusive. | |
| No | |
| No. There really is a lack of good published evidence. One problem, however, is that the synthesis does not include operational products within agencies (i.e., white papers, special studies). In the VA, for example, OQP have conducted internal analysis of clinical quality and patient satisfaction metrics and generally found no differences between patients residing in rural and urban areas. | The task was to develop a synthesis of the existing published peer-reviewed evidence base. We did, however, examine studies conducted by OQP and AHRQ, and have commented on the findings of those reports in our discussion. |
| No | |
| **3. Are there any published or unpublished studies that we may have overlooked?** | |
| Not that I am aware of. | |
| I realize the scope of his review was on published, peer-reviewed literature but reports issued by government agencies that have undergone internal review should perhaps be considered particularly for "high level" views of disparities. The AHRQ National Health Disparities Report for 2008-2010 are worth consulting. The VHA-published Hospital Report Cards for 2008-2010 are worth consulting. The VHA report cards include breakdown of our performance measurement system (including process and satisfaction results) by rural vs. urban residence. | As noted above, we have now examined studies conducted by OQP and AHRQ, and have commented on the findings of those reports in our discussion. |
| It would also be helpful to expand the scope beyond the three data sources used and include more hand searching (some was done). Inclusion of relevant dissertation research would be helpful. Assuring that negative findings are included (since there is publication bias) would strengthen the findings. | While we agree that information from well controlled studies that did not make it to publication because of negative findings would be informative, the systematic nature of the evidence based synthesis report precludes the use of non-peer reviewed literature. |
| None that I can think of. | |
| The library of articles on telehealth, including telephone management. | When we began the literature review for this report, a separate report was being developed to cover the telehealth literature. |

| REVIEWER COMMENT | RESPONSE |
|---|---|
| See comment above about operational products within agencies. Some of these results are available in the public domain such as Data.gov and on VA Websites. | See comments above. |
| This is a very complete review. | Thank you. |
| **4. Are there any clinical performance measures, programs, quality improvement measures, patient care services, or conferences that will be directly affected by this report? If so, please provide detail.** | Thank you – we will share the responses to this question with the people responsible for dissemination of the report. |
| No | . |
| OQP plans to use this evidence review to inform our own measurement systems and reports, and will be particularly careful in our use of risk adjustment procedures that may "adjust away" the impact of rurality. We are also working closely with the Office of Rural Health to create more robust indicators of rural health disparities and believe the partnership will be strengthened by this report. | |
| Results should influence a) findings presented at annual HSR&D national meetings and b) programs funded by the Office of Rural Health | |
| This report should be disseminated widely and used as the basis for creating an agenda for systematically closing gaps in both knowledge and practice. VA's various centers (e.g., VERCs and QUERI groups) can use this report to help focus their efforts and assure that their work is applicable to veterans in rural and highly rural areas. | |
| Not that I am aware of. | |
| This paper has the potential to significantly impact and direct future directions in rural health research and rural health clinical implementation and quality improvement efforts. | |
| **5. Please provide any recommendations on how this report can be revised to more directly address or assist implementation needs.** | |
| a. I recommend leaving out studies that you do not believe contribute. It becomes hard to pick up on the important, relevant findings when everything is presented. Several of the studies were of different provider types not urban/rural differences in health care in my opinion. I also think that more clearly weighting and emphasizing the studies that you believe really are valid and generalizable would improve this paper. | We have clarified study quality within the text and have added the final Confidence Score rating to our evidence tables to assist readers. |
| b. I think you should add a quality rating column to your evidence tables. It is hard to go back and forth. I would like to see good summary tables in the text when possible. | |
| You may be able to give more specific recommendations to policy makers, such as which definition of rurality to use, as well as specific advice on how to adjust for patient mix so as not to submerge important rural/urban disparities. | It is our belief that the convention to be used in studies for the categorization of population density cannot be determined by this review and likely will vary depending on the type of study being conducted. Similarly, case mix adjustment depends on the focus of the study (e.g., whether or not to adjust for travel distance) will vary depending on the focus of the study. |

Rural vs. Urban Ambulatory Health Care: A Systematic Review

Evidence-based Synthesis Program

| REVIEWER COMMENT | RESPONSE |
|---|---|
| It would be helpful if there were tables (similar to the ones presenting the strength of evidence) with a + or a – or a NS, indicating which studies found significant rural-urban differences in the main constructs examined. This would allow the reader to get a quick visual on how many and what proportion of studies found differences in diabetes outcomes, for example. | We have added '+' and '-' indicators to our tables to assist readers. |
| Section a beginning on page 49 seems out of place in a summary section. Perhaps it would fit better directly after page 45. | When we began this report, a separate systematic review was to be conducted on telehealth interventions. For this reason, we chose to NOT evaluate telehealth studies and to focus instead on other types of interventions. However, since that review was not conducted, we agree with reviewers that examining only non-telehealth interventions makes little sense and so we have excluded that section from the final report. |
| This is a very dense report with lots of information. I liked the way the authors categorized their review by both their main questions and by disease categories within those. Some specific comments/suggestions:<br><br>a. Spell out their search terms – saying standard search terms isn't enough<br>b. Specify that you used the VA definition in the intro when you say 40% of veterans are rural<br>c. Even though it's already very long, the review really does lack the whole piece on telehealth that the VA in particular uses to compensate for in-person ambulatory access deficits. At least need to explain why you left that out.<br>d. Since this is a VA report, it might be helpful to segregate VA and non-VA studies within each category, or at least put asterisks on VA studies to denote them. Even saying they looked at "veterans" doesn't say for sure they were looking at VA services, or even VA users.<br>e. In terms of interventions, I didn't see a section on that to be able to give feedback on. I assume this would be the place to include telehealth. This may call for a separate literature review to include all telehealth terms and not rely on "rural" "urban" terms to get at the articles they want.<br>f. The point about paucity of prospective (or even longitudinal but non-interventional) studies is really important. I think this is where HSR&D should make the point (to ORH) that improving care and access to rural veterans is not just about observing and recording what's out there, but about planning interventions and prospectively evaluating their effect on rural veteran's health and access. | We have clarified our methods and the reasons why a review of telehealth interventions were not included. The section on interventions was removed for the reasons noted above.<br><br>There were an insufficient number of studies conducted within VA to separate them. However, we specifically note VA studies when they were reviewed. |
| Inclusion of non-published results per above comments. Because of the complexity of the issues, report should strongly recommend thoughtful "risk adjusted" analysis | Implications for risk adjustment have since been emphasized in the report. |
| **Additional Comments:** | |
| The finding that continuity of care was reported for rural residents although there was no evidence that they were more likely to have a usual source of care seems incongruous | The distinction has now been clarified in the text. |
| "Among the findings were higher rates of invasive cancer related to lower rates of screening" – Please specify – did the findings really link these two? | Yes, for cervical and breast cancers as we note. |

Rural vs. Urban Ambulatory Health Care: A Systematic Review

Evidence-based Synthesis Program

| REVIEWER COMMENT | RESPONSE |
|---|---|
| "Potential interactions of rurality and race (and/or income) should be considered." – You might comment that this area of research (at least evaluating outcomes) is extremely prone to confounding eg. people may move to urban settings when ill/needing more health care or, people who chose rural locations might make other health care choices than those choosing an urban setting | This was noted in the discussion. |
| "It remains to be determined, however, whether the observed lower health quality of life among rural veterans is due to differences in disease prevalence, disparities in health care or both." Or, different people choose different locals to live in. it is more complex than this in my opinion | We agree, and further clarified this in the text. |
| Regarding the literature search strategy figure, do you think there would be any value in adding more arrows to the bottom box telling what category the papers fell into? | We feel this might increase confusion. |
| The Institute of Medicine definition of disparity does not include variation due to differences in access (IOM, 2003). -Not sure I agree with this statement. I thought the IOM focused on all differences in utilization that were not due to differences in need and preference. I would just drop this sentence and the next | The specific reference was clarified in the text. |
| It might be nice to rate the relevance of the evidence to veterans. Perhaps each summary could start with the VA study or state that no VA study exists. | We specifically indicated which studies focused on veterans. Since many veterans use non-VA care and many of those who use VA split their care between VA and community providers, all studies are potentially relevant to veterans. |
| Mental Health section: Two studies were missed from the Journal of Rural Health that I think are important. One is a VA study.

Cully JA, Jameson JP, Phillips LL, Kunik ME, Fortney JC. Use of Psychotherapy by Rural and Urban Veterans. Journal of Rural Health, 26(3): 225-233, 2010.

Fortney JC, Harman JS, Xu S, Dong F. The Association between Rural Residence and the Use, Type, and Quality of Depression Care, Journal of Rural Health,26(3): 205-213, 2010. | These studies were published after our March 2010 pull date. However, given their relevance we note their findings in the discussion. |
| This study found higher suicidality in rural versus urban: Rost, K., M. Zhang, et al. (1998). "Rural-urban differences in depression treatment and suicidality." Medical Care 36(7): 1098-1107. | This study, which was already included in the review, was added to the section covering suicidality. |
| Here are two papers showing that rurality is related to hospitalization rates for depression and schizophrenia:

Fortney J, Rushton G, Wood S, Zhang I, Xu S, Dong F, Rost K. Community-Level Risk Factors for Depression Hospitalizations. Administration and Policy in Mental Health and Mental Health Services Research, 34(4): 343-352, 2007

Fortney J, Xu S, Dong F. Community-Level Correlates of Hospitalizations for Persons with Schizophrenia , Psychiatric Services, 60(6): 772-778, 2009. | We included these per your recommendation; however, the methods used were only suggestive regarding reasons for differential hospitalization rates in rural vs. urban areas. |
| "Moreover, while rural residents were found to receive fewer MH services than urban residents in several studies, the clinical impact of this difference was unclear." - See this article: Fortney J. Rost K. and Zhang M. The Impact of Geographic Accessibility on the Intensity and Quality of Depression Treatment. Medical Care 37(9):884-893, 1999. | We have now included this article in our review. |

Rural vs. Urban Ambulatory Health Care: A Systematic Review

Evidence-based Synthesis Program

| REVIEWER COMMENT | RESPONSE |
|---|---|
| Regarding CBOCs and VAMCs This study is actually the better study, as it is quasi-experimental:<br><br>Fortney J, Maciejewski M, Warren J, and Burgess J. Does Improving Geographic Access to VA Primary Care Services Impact Patients' Patterns of Utilization and Costs? Inquiry, 42(1):29-42, 2005 | The relationship between CBOC placement and rurality is not uniform, which is why we did not include this interesting article in our review. |
| Travel Distance - There are actually lots and lots of travel distance articles which you didn't find because you were searching for rural vs urban studies. You might need to either drop this or expand your search. | We agree that our search terms did not allow us to comment sufficiently on this topic. |
| "There is some weak evidence that urban residents have a lower threshold for seeking mental health care than do rural residents" - I don't really believe this. Severity at intake is not different between rural and urban patients. | We are aware of no studies that actually asses provider availability and patient treatment attitudes and needs in urban and rural residents and then associate those differences with use of mental health services. |
| "As has been shown by others (Weeks, Wallace, 2008; Berke, 2009; Stern, 2010) the definition of rural that is used in a study has a significant impact on the findings and, consequently, the policy implications." - I would also reiterate that rural is a proxy for many different things (travel time, stigma, lack of insurance, etc.), and that the rural vs urban literature does not determine what underlying factors are driving the findings. | We have clarified this in the report. |
| "Because many factors are correlated with rurality, adjusting for all available covariates may lead to false conclusions regarding the association of rurality and study outcomes, and provide insufficient information for the development of healthcare policy. For most research questions, a more contextual analytic approach should be used." – Good observation! Might want to include this point in the executive summary. | Thank you for this recommendation. We have now done so. |
| Where possible use data / numbers (and indicate statistical significance, if appropriate) instead of phrases like, little difference, or increased rates etc. or give the page number where the specific data is found later in the document | We have tried to improve the clarity of findings in the report. |
| "However, all but one study found a greater frequency of unstaged cancer at the time of diagnosis in rural areas compared to urban areas." - I think it would be good to mention the outcomes (present or absence of data) on how this finding affects mortality | No information about the implications of unstaged disease for outcomes were made in the papers reviewed. The odds of unstaged disease was not a primary focus of the studies, but was an incidental finding. |
| "Moreover, health care systems operate locally and identifying areas where problems are greatest would help policy makers target areas that have the most need." - Rurality may very well be different in various parts of the country i.e. rural Alaska is different than rural Mississippi etc. | We think these differences have received very little attention. |

# APPENDIX C. EVIDENCE TABLES

## Appendix C, Table 1. Preventive Care/Ambulatory Care Sensitive Conditions

| Author, Year, Study Design | Study Population (Sample Size, Inclusion/Exclusion, Region/Nationwide) | Data Source, Year(s) (if applicable) Response Rate (if applicable) | Definition of Urban/Rural | Covariates | Confidence Score* | Results** |
|---|---|---|---|---|---|---|
| Casey, 2001[18] Cross-sectional | N = 130,452 respondents<br><br>Exclusion: respondents whose BRFSS records could not be linked to ARF data using county Federal Information Processing Standard (FIPS) codes<br><br>Nationwide | National data from the 1997 Behavioral Risk Factor Surveillance System (BRFSS) and the 1999 Area Resource File | Urban = Metropolitan Statistical Area (MSA)<br><br>Rural adjacent: nonmetropolitan county physically adjacent to metropolitan<br><br>Rural nonadjacent county | Age, gender, education, Income, race/ethnicity, insurance coverage, primary care physicians/1000 population, census region | High | Influenza vaccination in the past year for women ≥ 65 years old (-)<br><br>Pneumonia vaccination for women ≥ 65 years old (-) |
| Epstein, 2009[27] Cross-sectional | N = 1,508<br><br>Inclusion: stratified random sample of 200 women who gave birth to a live child 60-100 days before selection date<br><br>Oregon | 2003 Oregon Pregnancy Risk Assessment Monitoring System<br><br>Oregon Birth Certificate database<br><br>Response: 65.8% | Rural-Urban Commuting Area Codes: urban, large rural, or small/isolated rural | Age, marital status, education, Hispanic ethnicity, intended or unintended pregnancy, household income, questionnaire language | Low/Moderate | Late initiation of prenatal care (-)<br><br>Barriers to prenatal care initiation (-) |
| Laditka, 2009[28] Cross-sectional | N = 1,000 for analyses of children and adults <65 yrs; counties with ≥ 500 for analyses of adults 65+<br><br>Inclusion: counties with ≥<br><br>Colorado, Florida, Kentucky, Michigan, New York, North Carolina, South Carolina, and Washington | Hospital discharge data for 2002 from State Inpatient Databases (SIDS); Area Resource File (2002); U.S. Census Bureau; U.S. Census Bureau's Small Area Health Insurance Estimates | 2003 Urban Influence Codes (U.S. Department of Agriculture) with 7 levels from large metro to most rural | Hospital bed supply, hospitals with EDs, health maintenance organization penetration, presence of community health center or rural health center, race, education, population density, unemployment, state fixed effects | Moderate | Hospitalizations for ambulatory care sensitive conditions – ages 18 to 64 (+); R>U<br><br>Hospitalization for ambulatory care sensitive conditions – ages 65 and older (+); R>U |
| Saag, 1998[29] Cross-sectional | N = 787<br><br>Inclusion: home-dwelling elderly (age > 65 years), ≥ 1 of the indicator conditions, resident of state's 12 most rural and 10 most urban counties<br><br>Iowa | Population based phone survey evaluating six common chronic indicator conditions (arthritis, hypertension, cardiac disease, diabetes mellitus, peptic ulcer disease, and chronic obstructive pulmonary disease)<br><br>Response: 57% | U.S. Department of Agriculture continuum codes.<br><br>Urban: metro areas with > 250,000 residents<br><br>Rural: <2,500 residents in a single incorporated place and not adjacent to metro areas | Age, gender, education beyond high school, living on a farm, alcohol use, smoking in the past, medical advice needed in the past year, supplemental private insurance, medication coverage, Medicaid, VA clinic in the past year, Distance from physician, congregate meals, Use of Meals on Wheels, Homemaker service | Low | Continuity of care (seeing same physician) (+); R>U<br><br>Appointments with specialists (+); R>U<br><br>Perceived need for medical advice (+); R<U |

**Rural vs. Urban Ambulatory Health Care: A Systematic Review**

| Author, Year, Study Design | Study Population (Sample Size, Inclusion/Exclusion, Region/Nationwide) | Data Source, Year(s) (if applicable) Response Rate (if applicable) | Definition of Urban/Rural | Covariates | Confidence Score* | Results** |
|---|---|---|---|---|---|---|
| Schreiber, 1997[30]<br><br>Cross-sectional | N = 1,461 Zip Codes with population >300<br><br>New York | New York State Department of Public Health; U.S. Census Bureau 1990 | Six point urban-rural scale based on population, size of largest city/town, % of workforce that commutes outside the county; grouped to New York City area, upstate New York urban-suburban, and more remote rural | % of population in poverty, population density (population per square mile, % blacks, number of primary care physicians per 1,000 population), location of ZIP code (within 8 miles of hospital, within a health professional shortage area [HPSA]) | Low | Ambulatory Care Sensitive Conditions (ACSC) admissions:<br>a) increased as population density decreased within each of the 3 defined regions (+)<br>b) increased as percentage of black residents increased (+) except in the most rural group (-)<br>c) increased as number of primary care physicians per 1000 increased (+) |
| Zhang, 2000[19]<br><br>Cross-sectional | N = 4,051<br><br>Inclusion: men and women aged 65 or older<br><br>Nationwide | 1994 National Health Interview Survey (NHIS)<br><br>Overall response: 79.5% | U.S. Office of Management and Budget's (MSAs and non-MSAs) | Census region, education, household income, insurance status, overall health status | Moderate | Flu shots received in previous year (-) |

*See Methods section for explanation

**U=Urban; R=Rural; HR=Highly rural; F=Frontier; S=Suburban; (+)=difference statistically significant; (-)=difference not statistically significant

## Appendix C, Table 2. Cancer Screening

| Author, Year Study Design | Study Population (Sample Size, Inclusion/Exclusion, Region/Nationwide) | Data Source, Year(s) (if applicable) Response Rate (if applicable) | Definition of Urban/ Rural | Covariates | Confidence Score* | Results** |
|---|---|---|---|---|---|---|
| Brown K., 2009[20] Cross-sectional | N = 1,922 women (620 rural) Inclusion: Non-Hispanic whites and non-Hispanic black, age ≥40, reporting screening mammography or no mammography Tennessee | Behavioral Risk Factor Surveillance System (BRFSS) 2001 and 2003 | Rural-Urban Continuum Codes (RUCCs) – collapsed to 2 levels: rural or urban | Age, race/ethnicity, marital status, education, employment, health status, smoker, health insurance, personal health care provider | Moderate | Screening mammography utilization (-) |
| Casey, 2001[18] Cross-sectional | N = 130,452 respondents Exclusion: respondents whose BRFSS records could not be linked to ARF data using county Federal Information Processing Standard (FIPS) codes; California data on mammograms and Pap tests (state had modified wording of those questions) | National data from the 1997 Behavioral Risk Factor Surveillance System (BRFSS) and the 1999 Area Resource File | Urban = Metropolitan Statistical Area (MSA) Rural adjacent = nonmetropolitan county physically adjacent to metropolitan Rural nonadjacent county | Age, gender, education, income, race/ethnicity, insurance coverage, primary care physicians/1000 population, census region | High | Colon cancer screening for women and men age ≥50 (+); U>all R Cervical cancer screening for women age > 18 (+); U>all R Mammogram for women age ≥50 (+); U>non-adjacent R |
| Coughlin, 2008[23] Cross-sectional | N = 97,820 (Pap smears), 91,492 (mammography) Inclusion: reported county of residence Pap smears-women with known Pap test status, ≥18 yrs, no history of hysterectomy Mammography-women with known mammography screening status, ≥40 yrs Nationwide excluding Alaska, including District of Columbia | Behavioral Risk Factor Surveillance System (BRFSS) 2002 Area Resource Files (ARF) 2004 Census 2002 | US Department of Agriculture (USDA) RUCC collapsed to 3 levels: rural, suburban, metropolitan | Individual-level covariates (e.g., age, race, marital status, education, income, employment, health insurance, health status) and contextual covariates (e.g., residence, number of health centers per population, number of physicians per population) | High | Pap test in counties with <300 primary care providers per 100,000 women (+); U>R, U>S Pap test in counties with 300-500 physicians per 100,000 women (+); U>S Mammogram (+); U>R, S>R |
| Coughlin, 2004[22] Cross-sectional | N = 23,565 men and 37,847 women, age ≥ 50 yrs Nationwide | Behavioral Risk Factor Surveillance System (BRFSS) 1998-1999 | USDA RUCC collapsed to 3 levels: rural, suburban, metropolitan | Race/ethnicity, age, gender, education, health insurance, visit to physician in past year, health profile, shortage area | High | Fecal occult blood test in past year (+); U>R, S>R Sigmoidoscopy or colonoscopy in past 5 years (+); U>R |
| Coughlin, 2002[21] Cross-sectional | N = 108,326 women, age ≥ 40 yrs (mammography and clinical breast examination) N=131,813 women, age ≥ 18 yrs, with no history of hysterectomy (Pap testing) Nationwide | Behavioral Risk Factor Surveillance System (BRFSS) 1998-1999 | USDA Beale Codes collapsed to 3 levels: metropolitan, suburban, rural | Age, gender, race, education, number of people in household, health status, visit to physician in past year, marital status | High | Mammogram in past 2 years (+); U>R, U>S, S>R Pap test in past 3 years (+); U>R |

Rural vs. Urban Ambulatory Health Care: A Systematic Review

Evidence-based Synthesis Program

| Author, Year Study Design | Study Population (Sample Size, Inclusion/Exclusion, Region/Nationwide) | Data Source, Year(s) (if applicable) Response Rate (if applicable) | Definition of Urban/ Rural | Covariates | Confidence Score* | Results** |
|---|---|---|---|---|---|---|
| Kinney, 2006[24] Case-control | N = 558 cases and 952 controls (matched on race, age, and gender) Inclusion (cases): ages 50-80 yrs, pathologically confirmed invasive adenocarcinoma of colon North Carolina | Interviews (face-to-face) 1996-2000 Response: 72% (cases), 62% (controls) | U.S. Census Bureau 1990 standards Urban: Metropolitan Statistical Area (1 city with ≥50,000 or total metro area of ≥100,000) Rural: non-metro-politan | Age, race, gender, education, poverty index, recent colorectal cancer screening | Moderate | Colon cancer screening (NR); U>R# #Unadjusted analysis |
| Schootman, 1999[25] Cross-sectional | N = 7,200 women Inclusion: Primary breast or cervical carcinoma diagnosed 1991-95, non-institutionalized, ≥18 yrs old Iowa | Behavioral Risk Factor Surveillance System (BRFSS) 1996-97 Surveillance, Epidemiology, and End Results (SEER) 1991-95 Response: 39% | Based on number of residents per square mile; 5 levels <20, 20-29, 30-39, 40-99, or 100 or more res/mi²; urban=more than 100 res/mi² | Breast cancer screening model: income, having health insurance Cervical cancer screening model: education, age, income, having health insurance | Moderate | Breast cancer screening (+); U>R Cervical cancer screening (+); U>R |
| Stearns, 2000[26] Cross-sectional | N = 12,637 Inclusion: Medicare enrollee for whole year, living in household for whole year Nationwide | Medicare Current Beneficiary Survey (MCBS) 1993 | 1993 Urban Influence Codes (UIC); 9 categories collapsed to 5 for this study | Age, gender, race, Medicaid status, income, education, living arrangement, health status, functional status, provider supply | Moderate | Mammogram in last year (-) (except rural county with city of >10,000 < urban) Pap test in last year (-) |
| Zhang, 2000[19] Cross-sectional | N = 8,970 (Pap smears) 2,729 (mammography), 4,051 (flu shots) Inclusion: completed all three sections of NHIS Three services: Pap smears in past 3 years for women 18-65 yrs, mammogram in past 2 years for women 50-69 yrs, flu shot in past year for people ≥65 yrs Nationwide | U.S. National Health Interview Survey (NHIS) 1994 Response: 80% | Metropolitan Statistical Areas (MSA); urban county is within MSA; rural is all other non-metropolitan counties | Education, household income, health insurance status, Census region | Moderate | Pap smear (-) Mammogram (-) |

*See Methods section for explanation

**U=Urban; R=Rural; HR=Highly rural; F=Frontier; S=Suburban; (+)=difference statistically significant; (-)=difference not statistically significant; (NR)=significance not reported

## Appendix C, Table 3. Cancer Care

| Author, Year, Study Design | Study Population (Sample Size, Inclusion/Exclusion, Region/Nationwide) | Data Source, Year(s) (if applicable) Response Rate (if applicable) | Definition of Urban/Rural | Covariates | Confidence Score* | Results** |
|---|---|---|---|---|---|---|
| Chirumbole, 2009[36]<br><br>Cross-sectional | N = 10,414 cases (pancreatic), 56,767 (colorectal)<br><br>Inclusion: colorectal or pancreatic cancer<br><br>Pennsylvania | Pennsylvania Department of Health, Bureau of Health Statistics Research 2000–05<br><br>US Census Bureau 2000<br><br>American Medical Association Physician-Related Data Resources | US Census Bureau; grouped 67 counties into 22 Workforce Investment Areas (WIA); rurality variable was % of a WIA population that was rural | Age, gender, insurance status, education, poverty status, race, number of physicians per 100,000, ratio of oncology physicians to primary care physicians | Low | Later stage at diagnosis: Pancreatic (+); U>R<br><br>Colorectal (-) |
| Elliott, 2004[35]<br><br>Data collected as part of group-randomized trial of intervention directed at rural providers | N = 2,568 (1,463 or 57% rural)<br><br>Inclusion: pathologically confirmed incident cancers of breast, colon, rectum, lung, or prostate; age ≥18 yrs, resided and had primary care physician in one of 18 rural study communities, spoke English, accrued within 6 weeks of diagnosis<br><br>Lake Superior region (Minnesota, Wisconsin, Michigan) | Health Care Records 1992-97 | U.S. Census Bureau | Age, oncology consultation | Low/ Moderate | *Proportion of cases staged at diagnosis:*<br>(+); U>R for breast, non-small cell lung, and prostate cancer<br>(-); colorectal and small cell lung cancer<br>*Stage at diagnosis:*<br>(+); R>U for breast, colorectal, and non-small cell lung cancer<br>(-); small cell lung or prostate cancer<br>*Initial management score:*<br>(+); R<U for all cancers<br>*Clinical trial participation:*<br>(+); R<U for colorectal and prostate cancer<br>*Surveillance testing score:*<br>(+); R<U lower breast and colorectal cancer<br>(-); for lung and prostate cancer |
| Higginbotham, 2001[37]<br><br>Cross-sectional | N = 9,685 cancer cases<br><br>Inclusion: incident cancer cases (primary cancer site)<br><br>Mississippi | Mississippi State Department of Health Central Cancer Registry and Division of Vital Statistics 1996 | Census data: county with more than 50% rural designated as rural | Age | Moderate | Cancer incidence (-)<br><br>Cancer mortality (-)<br>Cancer staged at diagnosis :<br>(+); U>R, all sites<br>(+); U>R; women<br>(+); U>R; African Americans (except lung cancer)<br>Advanced stage at diagnosis<br>(+); R>U all sites and lung cancer |

**Rural vs. Urban Ambulatory Health Care: A Systematic Review**

| Author, Year, Study Design | Study Population (Sample Size, Inclusion/Exclusion, Region/Nationwide) | Data Source, Year(s) (if applicable) Response Rate (if applicable) | Definition of Urban/Rural | Covariates | Confidence Score* | Results** |
|---|---|---|---|---|---|---|
| Kinney, 2006[24]<br><br>Case-control | N = 558 cases and 952 controls (matched on race, age, and gender)<br><br>Inclusion (cases): ages 50-80 yrs, pathologically confirmed invasive adenocarcinoma of colon<br><br>North Carolina | Interviews (face-to-face) 1996-2000<br><br>Response: 72% (cases), 62% (controls) | U.S. Census Bureau, 1990<br><br>Urban: Metropolitan Statistical Area (1 city with ≥50,000 or total metro area of ≥100,000)<br><br>Rural: non-metropolitan | Age, race, gender, education, poverty index, sampling probabilities | Moderate | Colon cancer stage at diagnosis (-) |
| Loberiza, 2009[34]<br><br>Retrospective cohort | N = 2,330<br><br>Inclusion: lymphoma complete prognostic clinical data, residential ZIP code<br><br>Patients with lymphoma reported to the Nebraska Lymphoma Study Group (Nebraska and surrounding states) | University of Nebraska Medical Center Oncology Database 1982-2006 | Rural-Urban Commuting Area code; collapsed to 2 categories<br><br>Providers classified as university- or community-based | Median household income, distance traveled, year of treatment | Low/ Moderate | Risk of death (-); risk greater for rural community treated patients than urban or rural university treated patients; in high-risk subgroup risk higher for all groups relative to urban university treated<br><br>Advanced treatment (-); use was higher in University-treated compared to community treated regardless of residence<br><br>Death from primary lymphoma (+); R>U |
| McLafferty, 2009[39] | N = 150,794 cases<br><br>Inclusion: breast, colorectal, lung, or prostate cancer; staged cases<br><br>Illinois | Illinois State Cancer Registry 1998-2002<br><br>Surveillance, Epidemiology, and End Results (SEER) staging data | Rural-Urban Commuting Areas: modified to create Chicago city, Chicago suburb, other metropolitan, large town, and rural | Multiple models<br>1) unadjusted<br>2) age, race<br>3) socioeconomic and access variables based on zip code | Moderate | Risk of late stage diagnosis:<br>*Model 1* (+); city > all other regions for all 4 cancers (except lung cancer in suburb)<br>*Model 2* (+); city > all other regions for colorectal, breast (except city similar to most rural), and lung (except city similar to suburb) cancers; city > suburb (only) for prostate cancer<br>*Model 3* (+); city >other metro and large town for breast, city > large town for colorectal, and city >all regions except suburb for lung cancers |

Rural vs. Urban Ambulatory Health Care: A Systematic Review

Evidence-based Synthesis Program

| Author, Year, Study Design | Study Population (Sample Size, Inclusion/Exclusion, Region/Nationwide) | Data Source, Year(s) (if applicable) Response Rate (if applicable) | Definition of Urban/Rural | Covariates | Confidence Score* | Results** |
|---|---|---|---|---|---|---|
| McLaughlin, 2009[41] Nested case-control | N = 453 patients. Inclusion: continuous Medicaid enrollment, newly started on aromatase inhibitor or tamoxifen, hormone receptor-positive tumors, stage I-III breast cancer, started adjuvant hormonal monotherapy during study, female, ≥55 yrs, white or African American. North Carolina | Linked North Carolina Central Cancer Registry-Medicaid Claims data 2000-04 | US Census Bureau and US Department of Health and Human Services- urban or rural | Tumor size, type of surgery, race, type of provider and practice setting, admitted to hospital, admitted to nursing facility, receiving home health care, age | Low/ Moderate | Treatment with aromatase inhibitors (+); U>R |
| Paquette, 2007[38] Cross-sectional | N = 129,811 (colorectal), 161,479 (lung). Inclusion: all adults (≥20 yrs) in SEER database with primary colorectal or lung cancer. Nationwide | Surveillance, Epidemiology, and End Results (SEER) database (National Cancer Institute), 2000-03 | Rural-Urban Continuum Codes (RUCCs) – 9 levels collapsed to: rural (levels 7 and 9) or urban (levels 1 to 3) | Age, race, language isolation, gender, marital status, income | Moderate | Unstaged cancer rates: Colorectal (+); R>U Lung (+); R>U#. Stage IV at presentation: Colorectal (+); U>R Lung (+); U>R. #Unadjusted analysis |
| Sankara-narayanan, 2009[40] | N = 6,561 cases. Inclusion: incident colorectal cancer; age ≥19 yrs, no missing data in registry. Nebraska | Nebraska Cancer Registry 1998-2003. Surveillance, Epidemiology, and End Results (SEER) staging data | Office of Management and Budget (OMB) 2003 definitions: urban metropolitan, micropolitan nonmetropolitan, rural nonmetropolitan | Age, gender, race/ethnicity, marital status, education, income, insurance, anatomic site | Moderate/ High | Early stage at diagnosis (+); Micropolitan>R (metropolitan no different from rural) |
| Schootman, 1999[25] Cross-sectional | N = 7,200 women. Inclusion: primary breast or cervical carcinoma diagnosed 1991-95, non-institutionalized, ≥18 yrs old. Iowa | Behavioral Risk Factor Surveillance System (BRFSS) 1996-97. Surveillance, Epidemiology, and End Results (SEER) 1991-95. Response: 39% | Based on number of residents per square mile; 5 levels <20, 20-29, 30-39, 40-99, or 100 or more res/ mi²; urban=more than 100 res/mi² | Age | Moderate | In situ breast cancer rate (NR); R<U. Invasive cervical carcinoma (NR); R>U. Breast or cervical cancer mortality (-) |
| Schootman, 2001[42] Cross-sectional | N = 6,988 (502 [7%] rural). Inclusion: women, all ages, diagnosed with primary microscopically confirmed DCIS 1991-1996, treated with breast conserving surgery. 9 metropolitan areas and 5 states across U.S. | Surveillance, Epidemiology, and End Results (SEER) program. Area Resource File (ARF) | Metropolitan Statistical Area | SEER registry, year of diagnosis | Moderate | Receipt of radiation therapy: Age <65 yrs (+); R<U Age 65+ (-) |

Rural vs. Urban Ambulatory Health Care: A Systematic Review

Evidence-based Synthesis Program

| Author, Year, Study Design | Study Population (Sample Size, Inclusion/Exclusion, Region/Nationwide) | Data Source, Year(s) (if applicable) Response Rate (if applicable) | Definition of Urban/Rural | Covariates | Confidence Score* | Results** |
|---|---|---|---|---|---|---|
| Shugarman 2008[33] | N = 26,073 (84.2% urban, 6.3% large rural, 4.9% small rural, 4.6% isolated rural)<br><br>Inclusion: continuously enrolled Medicare beneficiaries, age 65+, first diagnosed cancer was lung cancer 1995-99<br><br>Exclusion: enrolled in managed care, end-stage renal disease, eligible for Medicare due to disability<br><br>14 registries nationwide | SEER data linked to Medicare claims<br><br>Area Resource File | Rural-urban commuting area (RUCA codes) – 30 codes collapsed to 4 categories: urban, large rural city, small rural town, isolated small rural town | Gender, race/ethnicity, age at diagnosis, median ZIP code income, comorbidities, number of subspecialists, number of hospitals, residing in health professional shortage area, residing in census tract with >15% non-fluent English speakers | Moderate | Mortality (-)<br><br>Unstaged at diagnosis (-)<br><br>Stage at diagnosis (-)<br><br>Number of subspecialists (+); R<U<br><br>Receipt of radiation therapy (trend); R<U |

*See Methods section for explanation

**U=Urban; R=Rural; HR=Highly rural; F=Frontier; S=Suburban; (+)=difference statistically significant; (-)=difference not statistically significant; (NR)=significance not reported

Rural vs. Urban Ambulatory Health Care: A Systematic Review

Evidence-based Synthesis Program

## Appendix C, Table 4. Diabetes/End Stage Renal Disease (ESRD)

| Author, Year, Study Design | Study Population (Sample Size, Inclusion/Exclusion, Region/Nationwide) | Data Source, Year(s) (if applicable) Response Rate (if applicable) | Definition of Urban/Rural | Covariates | Confidence Score* | Results** |
|---|---|---|---|---|---|---|
| Andrus, 2004[47] Non-RCT | N = 187 Inclusion: type II diabetes, two or more visits to their clinic in the past 12 months (Rural = 78, Urban = 109) Alabama | Medical records of patients seen in clinics between January and August 2001 Data collection took place Aug-Sept 2001 in Rural clinic; and Feb-March 2002 in urban clinic | Not defined other than rural family practice clinic was a "physician-owned private family practice clinic with one physician provider" and urban internal medicine clinic included five physicians specializing in internal medicine and one physician specializing in endocrinology | None | Very Low | Preventive care consistent with American Diabetes Association guidelines (NR); R<U# Blood pressure, lipid, and HbA1c goals met (NR); R<U# #Unadjusted analysis |
| Koopman, 2006[48] Cross-sectional | N = 947 Inclusion: US civilian, ≥20 years, non-institutionalized, participated in NHANES III: household adult, examination, and laboratory data files Exclusion: did not participate in all three parts of the survey Nationwide | Third National Health and Nutrition Examination Survey (NHANES III) 1988-1994 | Urban: MSA Rural: Non-MSA | Gender, age, BMI, perceived health status, income, insurance status, education, usual place of care, # times seeing physician in past year, duration of diabetes | Moderate | Undiagnosed diabetes (-) Uncontrolled BP (+); RHispanics>UHispanics Glycemic control (-) Cholesterol control (-) |
| Krishna, 2010[45] Cross-sectional | BRFSS (N = 441,351) MEPS (N = 48,428) Inclusion: age 18 and older Nationwide | Behavioral Risk Factor Surveillance System (BRFSS) 2001-2002; Medical Expenditure Panel Survey (MEPS) 2001-2002. | Urban: MSA Rural: Non-MSA | Age, BMI, insurance coverage, gender, race/ethnicity, education, region of country, income, personal physician | Moderate/ High | Prevalence of diabetes (+); R>U Compliance with diabetes care guidelines for eye exam, foot exam, diabetes education (+); R<U based on BRFSS (-); based on MEPS (eye and foot exam only) Compliance with guidelines for HbA1c test (-) |

73

Rural vs. Urban Ambulatory Health Care: A Systematic Review

Evidence-based Synthesis Program

| Author, Year, Study Design | Study Population (Sample Size, Inclusion/Exclusion, Region/Nationwide) | Data Source, Year(s) (if applicable) Response Rate (if applicable) | Definition of Urban/Rural | Covariates | Confidence Score* | Results** |
|---|---|---|---|---|---|---|
| Morden, 2010[49] Cross-sectional | N=11,688 Inclusion: Veterans with diabetes Nationwide | 2005 national Veterans Health Administration cardiometabolic quality of care random sample chart review SMITREC: VA Serious Mental Illness Treatment and Evaluation Center | RUCA categories RUCA 1: urban RUCA 2: large rural city/town RUCA 3: small/isolated rural town | Mental disorder diagnosis, RUCA (1-3), age, gender, race (black/non-black), marital status, substance abuse diagnosis, Charlson comorbidity index score, # VA outpatient visits, # visits to a VA community-based outpatient clinic, VA cost share category | Moderate/ High | LDL, foot exams, eye exams, renal testing, HbA1c, blood pressure (-) |
| O'Hare, 2006[44] Cross-sectional | N = 552,279 (and 4,363 dialysis facilities Inclusion: initiated dialysis between 1/1/95 and 12/31/02 and survived >90 days without transplant Nationwide | U.S. Renal Data System 2000 U.S. Census CMS Dialysis Facilities Compare database | Rural-Urban Commuting Area Codes (RUCA): Urban area Large Rural Area Small Rural Area Remote, Small Rural Area | Age, gender, comorbid conditions at start of dialysis, dialysis modality at 90 days; ZIP code per capita income and % >25 yrs with high school diploma Stratified for race/ethnicity | High | Survival (+); all R white non-Hispanic > U white non-Hispanic; remote small R white Hispanic < U white Hispanic; small R and remote small R black > U black Time to kidney transplant (+); all R white non-Hispanic > U white non-Hispanic; large R and small R black < U black; remote small R Native American > U Native American |
| Rosenblatt, 2001[50] Cross-sectional | N = 30,589 Inclusion: all fee-for-service Medicare (continuous coverage) patients, 65+ years, alive at the end of the 1994, 2+ physician encounters for diabetes care in 1994, all medical care in Washington Washington state | Medicare Part B claims data 1994 | RUCA subset: Urban Adjacent Large Rural Rural Remote Large Rural Adjacent Small Remote Small | Sociodemographic factors, comorbidities, provider specialty | Moderate | Glycated hemoglobin test (+); Adjacent large R<all other locations (+); Large remote > all others |
| Ward, 2009[48] Cross-sectional | N = 18,377 (from 1,681 ZIP codes with analysis by ZIP) Inclusion: age ≥ 20 years, treated incident end-stage renal disease (ESRD) attributed to diabetes or autosomal dominant polycystic kidney disease (ADPCKD) 1/1/01 to 6/30/04, California resident California | U.S. Renal Data System*, 2000 U.S. Census, California Office of Statewide Health Planning and Development*, U.S. Dept of Health and Human Services Health Resources* *1/1/01 to 6/30/04 | U.S.D.A Rural-Urban Commuting Area Codes; 10 levels collapsed to rural (codes 9, 10) or urban (codes 1-8) | Socioeconomic status (income, proportion with income <200% of poverty level, house value, rent, education, % college graduates), insurance status, hospitalization for hypoglycemic events, rural location | Low | Annual incidence of ESRD attributed to diabetes (-) Annual incidence of ESRD attributed to autosomal dominant polycystic kidney disease (-) |

| Author, Year, Study Design | Study Population (Sample Size, Inclusion/Exclusion, Region/Nationwide) | Data Source, Year(s) (if applicable) Response Rate (if applicable) | Definition of Urban/Rural | Covariates | Confidence Score* | Results** |
|---|---|---|---|---|---|---|
| Weingarten, 2006[51] Cohort | Inclusion: fee-for-service Medicare beneficiaries with diabetes, ages 18-75, enrolled for prior 12 months with ≥23 months of continuous Part B coverage, ≥ 1 inpatient or emergency visit or 2 outpatient visits ≥7 days apart<br><br>Exclusion: gestational diabetes, died during measurement period<br><br>Nationwide | CMS National Diabetes Database (Part of Medicare Health Care Quality Improvement Program) 1999-2001<br><br>Participants identified from Part A and Part B claims data | County codes from the Federal Information Processing Standards; based on urban-rural continuum codes – 9 codes collapsed to 3: Urban, Semi-rural (adjacent to metropolitan area), Rural (not adjacent) | Race (white/non-white), ethnicity (Hispanic/non-Hispanic), states (Census divisions) | Low | Indicator rate*<br>A. in 10 top performing states (many in northern and eastern regions of US): 1 of 10 SR<U, 3 of 10 SR>U; 2 of 10 R<U, 2 of 10 R>U<br>B. in 10 lowest performing states (many in south): 9 of 10 SR<U, 1 of 10 SR>U; 7 of 10 R<U, 1 of 10 R>U<br><br>*Indicator rate = Annual HbA1c measurement; Biennial lipid profile; Biennial eye exam |

*See Methods section for explanation

**U=Urban; R=Rural; SR=Semi-rural; (+)=difference statistically significant; (-)=difference not statistically significant; (NR)=significance not reported

Rural vs. Urban Ambulatory Health Care: A Systematic Review

Evidence-based Synthesis Program

## Appendix C, Table 5. Cardiovascular Disease

| Author, Year, Study Design | Study Population (Sample Size, Inclusion/Exclusion, Region/Nationwide) | Data Source, Year(s) (if applicable) Response Rate (if applicable) | Definition of Urban/Rural | Covariates | Confidence Score* | Results** |
|---|---|---|---|---|---|---|
| Colleran, 2007[55] Cross-sectional | N = 200 Inclusion: 50 + years old, seen more than once at the study sites (1 urban academic medical center, 1 rural community clinic) in the previous year New Mexico | Medical record review; randomly selected charts to include 50 patients with cardiovascular disease (CVD) (25 Hispanic, 25 non-Hispanic white) and 50 without CVD from each site | Not defined other than "urban academic medical center", "rural community clinic" | Age, gender, hypertension, diabetes, dyslipidemia, smoking status | Low | Standard medications for treatment of CVD (+); U>R[#] Cholesterol lowering medications (+); U>R[#] Attainment of blood pressure goal (+); U>R[#] Attainment of LDL goal (-)[#] [#]Unadjusted analysis |
| Dellasega, 1999[56] Case Reports | N = 32 Inclusion: Patients from tertiary care center serving 31 counties, 65+ years old, primary diagnosis a medical or surgical cardiac condition, cognitively intact, being discharged to home Pennsylvania | Patient medical records; phone survey post-discharge to 20 weeks Survey Response: 32/50 completed all five surveys (60%) | Pennsylvania Dept of Aging Rural Services Task Force seven designations: Philadelphia, Allegheny, urban, suburban, semi-urban, semi-rural, and rural (based on population density and proximity to major metropolitan area) | Age, gender, marital status, education, number of hospitalizations, severity of illness | Very Low | Number of medications at discharge and during follow-up (+); U>R with more fluctuations in medications in urban patients Number of cardiac medications at discharge and during follow-up (+); U>R General Health SF-36 scale (NR); R improved over time, U decreased over time |
| Hicks, 2010[53] Cross-sectional | N = 778 surveys Inclusion: Provider completed survey after patient encounter, non-pregnant adult with type 2 diabetes 26 practices in Colorado (13 urban; 13 rural) | Provider questionnaire, June 2003-May 2004 Response: not stated | Rural: community of fewer than 25,000 residents at least 32 km (20 mi) from a major metropolitan center | Age, gender, race, ethnicity, BP (near goal or uncontrolled), practice level, communication problems, income level, number of prescription medications | Moderate | Provider taking action if BP was poorly controlled (-) Number of medications (+); R>U |
| King, 2006[54] Cross-sectional | N = 300 Inclusion: outpatient, diagnosed hypertension (100 from an urban, a suburban, and a rural clinic) South Carolina | Medical record review; consecutive sample | Not defined other than "urban university family practice center", "suburban residency practice", "rural private practice" clinics | Age, race, gender, number of medications, number of visits in past 12 months, comorbidities | Very Low | Blood pressure control (+); R>U |

Rural vs. Urban Ambulatory Health Care: A Systematic Review

Evidence-based Synthesis Program

| Author, Year, Study Design | Study Population (Sample Size, Inclusion/Exclusion, Region/Nationwide) | Data Source, Year(s) (if applicable) Response Rate (if applicable) | Definition of Urban/Rural | Covariates | Confidence Score* | Results** |
|---|---|---|---|---|---|---|
| Morden, 2010[49]<br><br>Cross-sectional | N = 23,780<br><br>Inclusion: Veterans with hypertension (approximately 1/3 with mental disorder [MD])<br><br>Nationwide | 2005 national Veterans Health Administration cardiometabolic quality of care random sample chart review<br><br>SMITREC: VA Serious Mental Illness Treatment and Evaluation Center | RUCA categories<br>RUCA 1: urban<br>RUCA 2: large rural city/town<br>RUCA 3: small/isolated rural town | Mental disorder diagnosis, RUCA (1-3), age, gender, race (black/non-black), marital status, substance abuse diagnosis, Charlson comorbidity index score, # VA outpatient visits, # visits to a VA community-based outpatient clinic, VA cost share category | Moderate/ High | Blood pressure control (-) |

*See Methods section for explanation

**U=Urban; R=Rural; (+)=difference statistically significant; (-)=difference not statistically significant; (NR)=significance not reported

Rural vs. Urban Ambulatory Health Care: A Systematic Review

Evidence-based Synthesis Program

## Appendix C, Table 6. HIV/AIDS

| Author, Year, Study Design | Study Population (Sample Size, Inclusion/Exclusion, Region/Nationwide) | Data Source, Year(s) (if applicable) Response Rate (if applicable) | Definition of Urban/Rural | Covariates | Confidence Score* | Results** |
|---|---|---|---|---|---|---|
| Cohn, 2001[58] Cohort | N = 3,173 (367 rural) Inclusion: HIV-infected adults who received care from January through June, 1996 Contiguous United States | HIV Cost and Services Utilization Study (HCSUS) 1996; rural component | Urban: MSA or New England county metropolitan areas Rural: non-MSA Office of Budget and Management, 1992 | Age, gender, race, ethnicity, risk group behavior, education, insurance, household income, region of care, CD4 count, HIV provider type | Moderate/ High | Appointments with providers caring for more HIV-infected patients (+); urban care > rural care[#] Use of pneumocystis carinii pneumonia medication (+); urban care > rural care[#] Use of highly-active antiretroviral therapy (HAART) (+); urban care > rural care |
| Napravnik, 2006[59] Cross-sectional | N = 1,404 Inclusion: 18+ years, attended ≥ 1 clinic appointment at a Univ. of North Carolina HIV clinic between 1/1/2000 and 12/31/2002 Southeastern United States (predominantly North Carolina) | Patient medical records from the University of North Carolina HIV outpatient clinic | Rural: MSA with < 50,000 inhabitants | Age, gender, race/ethnicity, insurance status, distance to clinic, clinical AIDS diagnosis, CD4 cell count, time since entry into HIV care | Moderate | Average number of clinic visits per year (-)[#] |
| Schur, 2002[60] Cohort | N = 275 rural patients Inclusions: HIV infected adults, receiving care from sampled providers (≥ 1 visit in early 1996) Exclusions: patients seen by military, prison, or emergency department providers Contiguous United States | HIV Cost and Services Utilization Study (HCSUS) 1996 American Medical Association MasterFile of physicians | Urban: MSA Rural: non-MSA Office of Budget and Management, 1992 | Age, gender, race/ethnicity, risk group, clinical stage, annual income, insurance status, CD4 count | Moderate | 73.6% of rural residents received HIV care in urban setting[#] Older patients more likely to receive care in rural area (+)[#] |
| Whyte, 1992[57] Cohort | N = 308 AIDs cases Inclusion: female residents of Georgia aged 13 and older at time of diagnosis whose cases were reported by 12/31/90 Georgia | Centers for Disease Control and Prevention (1983-1990) Office of Vital Statistics (Georgia), March 1991 | Metro Atl: residents of 8 counties of metropolitan Atlanta Other Areas: residents of remaining counties | Race, mean age, mode of infection | Very Low | Median survival time (+); Metro>Other[#] Probability of surviving 90 days (+); Metro>Other[#] |

*See Methods section for explanation
**U=Urban; R=Rural; (+)=difference statistically significant; (-)=difference not statistically significant; (NR)=significance not reported
[#]Unadjusted results

Rural vs. Urban Ambulatory Health Care: A Systematic Review

Evidence-based Synthesis Program

## Appendix C, Table 7. Neurologic Conditions

| Author, Year, Study Design | Study Population (Sample Size, Inclusion/Exclusion, Region/Nationwide) | Data Source, Year(s) (if applicable) Response Rate (if applicable) | Definition of Urban/Rural | Covariates | Confidence Score* | Results** |
|---|---|---|---|---|---|---|
| Buchanan, 2006b[62] Cohort | N = 1,518. Inclusion: Member of the National Multiple Sclerosis (MS) Society. Exclusion: none. Nationwide | Phone interview, Oct 2004 – Jan 2005. Response: 31% | Urban: Metropolitan Statistical Area (MSA). Adjacent Rural Area: <50 miles from MSA. More Remote Rural Area: >50 miles from MSA | None | Very Low | Saw neurologist in past year (+); U>MRR#. Wanted to see neurologist but did not (+); MRR>U, AR>U#. Majority of MS care from primary care physician (+); MRR>U# |
| Buchanan, 2006a[61] Cohort | N = 1,518. Inclusion: Member of the National Multiple Sclerosis Society. Exclusion: none. Nationwide | Phone interview, Oct 2004 – Jan 2005. Response: 31% | Urban: Metropolitan Statistical Area (MSA). Adjacent Rural Area: <50 miles from MSA. More Remote Rural Area: >50 miles from MSA | None | Low/ Very Low | Taking disease-modifying medications (+); U>MRR#. Discontinued disease-modifying medications because of other medical side effects(+); AR>U#. Discontinued disease-modifying medications because of out-of-pocket expense (+); AR>U# |
| Buchanan, 2006c[63] Cohort | N = 1,518. Inclusion: Member of the National Multiple Sclerosis Society. Exclusion: none. Nationwide | Phone interview, Oct 2004 – Jan 2005. Response: 31% | Urban: Metropolitan Statistical Area (MSA). Adjacent Rural Area: <50 miles from MSA. More Remote Rural Area: >50 miles from MSA | None | Very Low | Need for mental health care in past 12 months (+); AR<U, MRR<U#. No insurance coverage for mental health care (+); AR>U, MRR>U#. No providers in area or too far to visit (+); AR>U# |
| Wilson, 2009[66] Cross-sectional | N = 1,427 counties or county sets (contiguous, single state sets of counties merged to achieve population >50,000). Inclusion: all US counties or county sets except Alaska, Hawaii, and 12 cities with changes in county definitions between 1980 and 2000. Nationwide | Numbers of rehabilitation therapists (physical [PT] or occupational [OT] therapists, speech-language pathologists [SLP]) from 1980 and 1990 ARF and 2000 EEO. Health Professional Shortage Area Data | US Office of Management and Budget (OMB) – metropolitan (metro): central county with ≥1 urbanized area and outlying counties economically tied to core county | None | Moderate/ High | PTs, OTs, or SLPs per 100,000 residents (NR); U>R#. PTs, OTs, or SLPs per 100,000 residents (NR); Non-shortage area > partial or total shortage area# |

Rural vs. Urban Ambulatory Health Care: A Systematic Review

Evidence-based Synthesis Program

| Author, Year, Study Design | Study Population (Sample Size, Inclusion/Exclusion, Region/Nationwide) | Data Source, Year(s) (if applicable) Response Rate (if applicable) | Definition of Urban/Rural | Covariates | Confidence Score* | Results** |
|---|---|---|---|---|---|---|
| Johnstone, 2002[65]<br><br>Cross-sectional | Data on numbers of providers of services to people with traumatic brain injury<br><br>Missouri | U.S. Census Bureau, 2000; Office of Social and Economic Data Analysis, 2000; Rural Policy Research Institute, 2000; Missouri State Board of Registration for the Healing Arts, 1999; American Board of Professional Psychology; Missouri Brain Injury Association, 2000 | Office of Management and Budget (OMB) designations of Metropolitan and Non-metropolitan (MSA or non-MSA) | None | Moderate/High | Physicians (NR); U>R[#]<br>Physiatrists (NR); U>R[#]<br>Nurses (NR); U=R[#]<br>Rehabilitation Therapists (NR) U>R[#]<br>Mental Health (NR); U>R[#] |
| Schootman and Fuortes, 1999[64]<br><br>Cross-sectional | N = 292 patients age 18+ years with TBI sustained July–Dec 1996<br><br>Iowa | Survey sent to persons identified through the Iowa Central Registry for Brain and Spinal Cord Injuries, January, 1998<br><br>Response: 57.4% (292 is subset – those 18 years and older) | Population density (residents/square mile) – 5 levels<br><br><20, 20-29, 30-39, 40-99, 100+ | Injury severity, age, gender, type of respondent (injured person vs. proxy), inability to see a doctor because of cost | Low | Functional dependence (+); most urban > non-urban<br><br>Perceived need for services (-) |

*See Methods section for explanation
**U=Urban; R=Rural; MRR=More Remote Rural; AR=Adjacent Rural; (+)=difference statistically significant; (-)=difference not statistically significant; (NR)=significance not reported
#Unadjusted analysis

Rural vs. Urban Ambulatory Health Care: A Systematic Review

Evidence-based Synthesis Program

## Appendix C, Table 8. Mental Health

### Severe Mental Health

| Author, Year, Study Design | Study Population (Sample Size, Inclusion/Exclusion, Region/Nationwide) | Data Source, Year(s) (if applicable) Response Rate (if applicable) | Definition of Urban/Rural | Covariates | Confidence Score* | Results** |
|---|---|---|---|---|---|---|
| Farrell, 1996[72] Cross-sectional | N = 4,930 Inclusion: adults discharged from 8 public psychiatric hospitals to 1 of 40 community mental health centers (CMHC, 23 rural, 17 urban) in 1992 Virginia | Questionnaire (completed by CMHC staff), 1992 Inpatient Database Questionnaire completion rate: 97% (94% linked to database) | State mental health authority definition - rural is <120 people/ sq mi | None | Moderate | Continuity of care (+); R>U as indicated by a. CMHC had record of discharge, b. CMHC contacted patient during hospitalization, c. patient and CMHC had contact after discharge, d. CMHC provided face-to-face services, and e. composite score# #Unadjusted analysis |
| Fischer, 2008[73] Cohort | N = 258 (121 or 47% rural; included veterans) Inclusion: ages 18-67, schizophrenia, mental health service utilization records available for at least 18 months Arkansas | Interviews with patients (consumers) and family, friends, or providers who knew patient well (informants) 1992-99 | Office of Management and Budget – Urban: Metropolitan Statistical Area (MSA) Rural: non-MSA | Insight into illness, cognitive functioning, age, gender, ethnicity | Moderate | Irregular vs. regular outpatient mental health service use (+); R>U Comorbid substance abuse effect on mental health service use (+); less effect on patients with family support at least weekly |
| Mohamed, 2009[75] Cohort | N = 5,221 veterans (4,373 urban) Inclusion: participant in mental health intensive case management (MHICM) program Nationwide | Clinical process assessments by MHICM staff after veteran's 1st 6 months in MHICM program, FY2000-FY2005 VA Outpatient Encounter File | Rural-Urban Commuting Codes – 4-groups: urban (U), large rural city (LR), small rural town (SR), or isolated rural (R) community | None | Moderate | Patient contact (+); R<U# Receipt of services (+); all R<U Psychotherapy, substance abuse treatment, crisis intervention, medication management, screening or care for medical problems, rehabilitation, vocational support, housing support # #Unadjusted analysis |
| Rost & Owen, 1998[76] Cohort NOTE: telephone interviews with randomly selected adults in 11,078 households; 998 screened positive for depression | N = 54 (46 with 12 month follow-up) Inclusion: ≥18 yrs; screened positive for depression (telephone); not bereaved, manic, or acutely suicidal; lifetime mania identified in face-to-face interviews Arkansas | Telephone and face-to-face interviews 1992-93 Response: 85% of eligible after face-to-face interview with complete data (interview at 1 yr) | Urban: Metropolitan Statistical Area (MSA) Rural: non-MSA | Age, gender, education, health insurance, marital status, minority status, income, recent manic symptoms, severity of depression, previous psychiatric hospitalizations, recent drug/alcohol problems, psychiatric co-morbidity, physical condition. | Low | During 12 month follow-up: a. any non-acute mental health service (-) b. seen in general medical setting only (+); R>U c. any acute services for physical or mental health (+); R>U d. suicide attempt (-) e. manic episode (+); R>U f. depressive symptoms (-) |

Rural vs. Urban Ambulatory Health Care: A Systematic Review

| Author, Year, Study Design | Study Population (Sample Size, Inclusion/Exclusion, Region/Nationwide) | Data Source, Year(s) (if applicable) Response Rate (if applicable) | Definition of Urban/Rural | Covariates | Confidence Score* | Results** |
|---|---|---|---|---|---|---|
| **Hospitalization** | | | | | | |
| Fortney 2007[70] Cross-sectional | N = 811 counties Inclusion: 551, 529 depression related hospitalizations, age 20+ 14 states nationwide | Statewide Inpatient Database (SID), 2000 Census Bureau Dept. of Agriculture Health Resources and Services Administration | Urban Influence Codes (UIC) – 12 categories | Ethnicity, poverty level, education, income, employment, housing stress, county economy source, number of providers, number of hospital beds, penetration rate of HMOs, shortage area, geographic location | Low/ Moderate | Hospitalization rate (+); most U>all other UIC categories (5 comparisons were significant) |
| Fortney 2009[71] Cross-sectional | N = 811 counties Inclusion: 1443,107 schizophrenia related hospitalizations, age 20+ 14 states nationwide | Statewide Inpatient Database (SID), 2000 Census Bureau Dept. of Agriculture Health Resources and Services Administration | Urban Influence Codes – 12 categories U.S. Office of Management and Budget – MSA/non-MSA | Ethnicity, poverty level, education, income, employment, housing stress, county economy source, providers, hospital beds, penetration rate of HMOs, shortage area, geographic location | Low/ Moderate | Hospitalization rate (+);most U>all other UIC categories (8 comparisons were significant) |
| **Depression** | | | | | | |
| Fortney, 1999[74] Cohort | N = 106 of original 470 with depression visit in 6 months after baseline interview, complete data set, and provider in Arkansas (see Rost 1999) Arkansas | See Rost 1999 Records from providers, insurers, and pharmacies identified Geocoded addresses for travel time | Used travel time | Age, gender, ethnicity, employment status, education, severity of depression, physical and psychiatric comorbidities, insurance coverage, treatment sector | Low/ Moderate | Number of visits (+); increased travel time associated with fewer visits. Guideline concordant treatment (+); increased travel time associated with reduced odds of guideline concordant treatment |
| Rost, 2007[78] Cross-sectional (combining data from 2 studies) | N = 1,455 (304 rural) Inclusion: primary care patients with depression (excluded schizophrenia and bipolar disorder) 11 states | 2 studies in Quality Improvement for Depression database (through 1999): 1) Partners in Care (PIC), 46 practices (3 rural), 5 states (35% agreed to participate; follow-up 89% at 2 yr) 2) Quality Enhancement by Strategic Teaming (QuEST), 12 practices (4 rural), 10 states (73% agreed to participate, follow-up 70% at 2 yr) | Practices designated as urban (MSA) or rural (non-MSA) | Age, gender, minority status, education, marital status, employment, depression, psychiatric or physical comorbidity, antidepressant use, social support, stressful life events | Low | Baseline characteristics: a. use of outpatient care (specialty, medical) - past 6 mos (-)# b. antidepressant use -past 6 mos (-)# c. any hospitalization - past 6 mos (-)# Hospitalization for physical problems in 6 months after baseline (+); R>U whether or not they received specialty care during those 6 months Hospitalization for emotional problems (+); R>U at 18 months #Unadjusted analysis |

Rural vs. Urban Ambulatory Health Care: A Systematic Review

Evidence-based Synthesis Program

| Author, Year, Study Design | Study Population (Sample Size, Inclusion/Exclusion, Region/Nationwide) | Data Source, Year(s) (if applicable) Response Rate (if applicable) | Definition of Urban/Rural | Covariates | Confidence Score* | Results** |
|---|---|---|---|---|---|---|
| Rost, 1999[77] Cross-sectional NOTE: telephone interviews with randomly selected adults in 11,078 households; 998 screened positive for depression | N = 434 (286 rural) of original 470 with 12 month data Inclusion: ≥18 yrs; screened positive for depression (both telephone and face-to-face interviews); not bereaved, manic, or acutely suicidal Arkansas | Telephone and face-to-face interviews 1992-93 Response: 74% of eligible after screening agreed to face-to-face interview; 92% with complete data | Census data 1990, rural defined as non-metropolitan | Age, gender, education, health insurance, marital status, minority status, employment status, income, living alone, health insurance, severity of depression, physical and psychiatric comorbidity | Moderate | Any outpatient treatment for depression (-) Type of outpatient treatment for depression (-) Quality of outpatient depression treatment (-) Outpatient specialty care visits for depression (+); R<U Outpatient general medicine visits for depression (-) Change in depression severity (-) Hospitalization for physical problems (+); R>U Hospitalization for mental health problems (-) |
| Rost & Zhang, 1998[69] Cross-sectional | See Rost 1999 | See Rost, 1999 | Census data 1990, rural defined as non-metropolitan | See Rost, 1999 | Moderate | Outpatient services for physical problems (-) Outpatient services for mental health other than depression (-) Hospitalizations for physical or mental health problems 1-6 months after baseline (+); R>U Hospitalizations in months 7-12 (-) Suicide attempts (+); R>U |
| *Post Traumatic Stress Disorder (PTSD)* | | | | | | |
| Elhai, 2004[79] Cross-sectional | N = 100 veterans (52 rural) Inclusion: male, diagnosed with PTSD at outpatient clinic Southeastern United States | Medical chart review (date not reported) | U.S. Census data 1990 | Service use adjusted for distance and driving time | Very Low | Service use (PTSD clinic, primary care, and specialty care visits) within 1 year after initial PTSD evaluation (-) Dissociative Experiences Scale score (+); R>U MMPI-2 clinical scales (-) |

**Rural vs. Urban Ambulatory Health Care: A Systematic Review**

| Author, Year, Study Design | Study Population (Sample Size, Inclusion/Exclusion, Region/Nationwide) | Data Source, Year(s) (if applicable) Response Rate (if applicable) | Definition of Urban/Rural | Covariates | Confidence Score* | Results** |
|---|---|---|---|---|---|---|
| *Substance Abuse* | | | | | | |
| Booth, 2000[80] Cohort | N = 733 Inclusion: current adult drinkers (18+) who met DSM-IV criteria for alcohol abuse or dependence in the past year or were at risk for meeting DSM-IV diagnostic criteria in the following year Six southern states (AL, AR, GA, LA, MS, TN) | Telephone interview Response: 76% (baseline); 90% and 82% of baseline completed interview at 6 and 12 months, respectively | Census Bureau definitions of MSA; rural is non-MSA | Gender, ethnicity, age, income, health insurance, average time to provider, days to see MD for advice about drinking, acceptability of treatment, social support, alcohol abuse (past 6 months), alcohol dependence (past 6 months), lifetime drug use, Axis I DIS diagnosis (past 6 months), antisocial personality disorder, social consequences of drinking, negative life events, chronic medical problems, prior treatment for alcohol problems | Moderate/ High | Twelve month alcoholism treatment use (-) |
| Fortney et al., 1995[84] Cohort | N = 4,621 Inclusion: adult (18+) male veterans completing inpatient alcoholism treatment at VA Alcohol Dependency Treatment Program (ADTP) 33 VA inpatient ADTPs | VA Patient Treatment File, 1987 | Small community (outside an MSA); metropolitan area (MSAs with < 3 million inhabitants); large metropolitan area (MSAs with > 3 million inhabitants) | Distance to VA medical center, age, marital status, illness severity, race | Moderate | Attendance at outpatient appointment for alcoholism treatment 30 days after discharge from inpatient ADTP (+); small community > metropolitan, large metropolitan < metropolitan |
| Grant, 1996[81] Cross-sectional | N = 42,862 Inclusion: non-institutionalized adults (18+) Nationwide | National Longitudinal Alcohol Epidemiological Survey, 1992 Response: 97.4% (person); 91.9% (household) | Not provided | Gender, age, ethnicity, education, marital status, family history of alcoholism, past alcohol disorder and treatment, health insurance, employment, income, children < 14 at home, spouse/ partner with alcoholism, onset and severity of alcoholism, daily alcohol intake, major depression, comorbid drug use disorder; illicit drug use in past year | Moderate | Odds of entering treatment in the past year for drinking-related problems (-) |

Rural vs. Urban Ambulatory Health Care: A Systematic Review

Evidence-based Synthesis Program

| Author, Year, Study Design | Study Population (Sample Size, Inclusion/Exclusion, Region/Nationwide) | Data Source, Year(s) (if applicable) Response Rate (if applicable) | Definition of Urban/Rural | Covariates | Confidence Score* | Results** |
|---|---|---|---|---|---|---|
| Metsch & McCoy, 1999[82] Cross-sectional | N = 2,222 Inclusion: age 18+, self-reported drug use ≤30 days prior to recruitment; no active drug treatment 30 days prior to intake Two sites in Florida: Miami (urban) and Immokalee (rural) | In-person interview Response: not reported | Not defined Immokalee characterized as an unincorporated area known for agriculture and cattle industries | None | Low/ Moderate | Ever in drug-user treatment (+); U>R# Length of prior treatment (+); U>R# Treatment in past 24 months (+); U>R# Attempted but unable to get treatment in past 12 months (+); U>R# Of those using treatment, use of outpatient treatment (–)# #Unadjusted analysis |
| Robertson & Donnermeyer, 1997[83] Correlational | N = 3,629 (497 who used an illegal substance in the past year) Inclusion: age 21+, non-institutionalized, living in residential type of interest Nationwide | National Household Survey on Drug Abuse, 1991 Response: not reported | Rural defined as places with <2,500 inhabitants outside of or not next to urban areas (1980 Census) 3 residential types: metropolitan-rural (rural area within MSAs); non-metropolitan-rural; non-metropolitan-urban | NONE???? For this outcome | Low | 5.6% of nonmetropolitan-rural drug users sought treatment compared with 6.6% of the remaining respondents |
| **Suicide** | | | | | | |
| Fiske, 2005[68] Cross-sectional | N = 41 county clusters (counties of <100,000 grouped with neighboring counties) California (all counties) | California Departments of a. Health Service, Center for Health Statistics, 1993-2001 (odd years) b. Finance (population data) c. Consumer Affairs (providers) | U.S. Census Bureau; urbanicity of county based on proportion of county residents living in an urbanized area or town with population of ≥2,500 | Age | Low | Suicide rate (+); R>U Interaction between urbanicity and number of providers (–) (no association with suicide rate) |
| Gibbons, 2005[67] Cross-sectional | N = 91,673 Inclusion: all individuals who committed suicide Nationwide | National Vital Statistics (CDC) 1996-98 (suicide rates) IMS Health, Inc (antidepressant medication prescriptions) | Based on county population | Model 1: Age, gender, race Model 2: Added income Model 3: Added county mean drug prescription for each class of drugs | Low | Suicide rate (NR); smaller population counties>larger population counties Ratio of non-tricyclic antidepressants to tricyclic antidepressants (NR); larger population counties>smaller population counties |

**Rural vs. Urban Ambulatory Health Care: A Systematic Review**

| Author, Year, Study Design | Study Population (Sample Size, Inclusion/Exclusion, Region/Nationwide) | Data Source, Year(s) (if applicable) Response Rate (if applicable) | Definition of Urban/Rural | Covariates | Confidence Score* | Results** |
|---|---|---|---|---|---|---|
| *Utilization* | | | | | | |
| Hauenstein, 2006[87]<br><br>Cross-sectional | N = 32,319<br><br>Inclusion: civilian, non-institutionalized, 18-64 yrs<br><br>Nationwide | Medical Expenditure Panel Survey (MEPS), 1996-2000 data<br><br>Response: 73%-78% (varied by panel) | Rural-Urban Continuum Codes 1994; collapsed to metropolitan, non-metropolitan least rural, or non-metropolitan most rural | Gender, age, income-to-needs ratio, schooling, geographic region, mental health, physical health, marital status, number of children, usual source of care, insurance type, year | Moderate | Any mental health visit (+); U>most R and least R>most R for women<br><br>Specialized mental health visit (+) U>most R for women and men |
| Petterson, 2009[86]<br><br>Cross-sectional | N = 36,288<br><br>Inclusion: civilian, non-institutionalized, ≥18 yrs; non-Hispanic white, African American, Mexican American<br><br>Nationwide | Medical Expenditure Panel Survey (MEPS) 1996-2000 data<br><br>Response: 73%-78% (varied by panel) | Rural-Urban Continuum Codes 1994; collapsed to metropolitan, non-metropolitan least rural, or non-metropolitan most rural | Self-reported mental and physical health, gender, age, education, employment status, marital status, income-to-needs ratio, health insurance | Moderate | Receipt of any mental health service:<br>(+): African American < non-Hispanic white in any location<br>(+): Mexican American < non-Hispanic white, urban and least rural non-MSA only<br>Receipt of specialty mental health service:<br>(+) African American < non-Hispanic white in urban and least rural locations<br>(+) Mexican American <non-Hispanic white in Urban location only |
| Petterson, 2003[85]<br><br>Cross-sectional | N = 2,381<br><br>Inclusion: ≥ 1 visit of any mental health treatment during calendar year; civilian, non-institutionalized, 18-64 yrs<br><br>Nationwide | Medical Expenditure Panel Survey (MEPS) 1996-98 data<br><br>Response: 78% | Rural-Urban Continuum Codes 1993; collapsed to metropolitan or non-metropolitan | Gender, race/ethnicity, age, education, employment status, marital status, income-to-needs ratio, health insurance, mental health, physical health | Moderate | Any or specialized mental health visit:<br>(+): U>R if reported mental health was good or fair#<br>(-) if reported mental health was poor#<br><br>Mental health care use (-): trend for U>R<br>Ever hospitalized in calendar year (-)<br>Ever saw a medical doctor (-)<br>Primarily saw a medical doctor (-)<br><br>#Unadjusted analysis |

Rural vs. Urban Ambulatory Health Care: A Systematic Review

Evidence-based Synthesis Program

| Author, Year, Study Design | Study Population (Sample Size, Inclusion/Exclusion, Region/Nationwide) | Data Source, Year(s) (if applicable) Response Rate (if applicable) | Definition of Urban/Rural | Covariates | Confidence Score* | Results** |
|---|---|---|---|---|---|---|
| Wang, 2005[88] Cross-sectional | N = 9,282 (interviewed) Inclusion: ages 18+, English speaking Nationwide | National Comorbidity Survey Replication (NCS-R), 2001-2003 (face-to-face interviews) Response: 71% | U.S. Census Bureau, 2000; large (≥ 2 million) and small central city, large (≥ 2 million) and small suburbs or central city, adjacent area, rural area | Age, gender, race/ethnicity, education, marital status, family income, health insurance | Moderate/ High | Odds of receiving any mental health treatment in prior 12 months (+); rural<all non-rural  Odds of receiving specialty mental health treatment in prior 12 months (+); rural<all non-rural except suburb <2 million  Mental health treatment adequacy:  (+); rural>all non-rural for mental health specialty treatment (-); any service use, general medical, and non-health care treatment |

*See Methods section for explanation

**U=Urban; R=Rural; (+)=difference statistically significant; (-)=difference not statistically significant; (NR)=statistical significance not reported

## Appendix C, Table 9. Use of Medication

| Author, Year, Study Design | Characteristics of Study Population (Sample Size, Inclusion/Exclusion, Region of United States) | Data Source and Year(s) of Sampling (if applicable) Response rate (if applicable) | Definition of Urban/Rural | Covariates | Confidence Score* | Results** |
|---|---|---|---|---|---|---|
| Dellasega, 1999[56] Prospective/Longitudinal | N = 32 Elderly patients admitted to a large tertiary care center for cardiac condition. Specific inclusion criteria: 1) 65 or older; 2) has medical or surgical cardiac condition as primary diagnosis; 3) cognitively intact; 4) being discharged from hospital Pennsylvania | Medical records and telephone interviews Response rate: 50% | Seven-level county designations established by the Pennsylvania Department of Aging Rural Services Task Force merged into two categories (i.e., rural vs. urban) | Age, gender, severity of illness | Low | Number of medications (+); U>R |
| Fillenbuam, 1993[89] Correlational | N = 3,973 Individuals 65 or older who are identified as black or white Piedmont area of North Carolina | Duke Established Populations for Epidemiologic Studies of the Elderly, 1986-1987 Response rate: 80.3% (black); 87.2% white | U.S. Census Bureau Definition | Gender, marital status, age, education, functional status, medical status, self-rated health, number of medical visits in past year, continuity of care, overnight hospitalization in past year, insurance status, income | Low/Moderate | Medication use - elderly whites (+);U>R Medication use - elderly blacks (-) |
| Hanlon, 1996[90] Cross-sectional | N = 4,110 Individuals 65 or older who identify as black or white Piedmont area of North Carolina | Duke Established Populations for Epidemiologic Studies of the Elderly, 1986-1987 Response rate: 80.3% (black); 87.2% white | U.S. Census Bureau Definition | Age, race, gender, education, functional status, number of functional limitations, chronic disease status, number of health visits in past year, hospitalization in past year, continuity of care, Medicaid status | Low/Moderate | Prescription medication use (+); U>R Number of non-prescription medications (+); U>R Use of non-prescription medications (-) |
| Lago, 1993[91] Cross-sectional | N = 18,641 Elderly enrolled in the Pennsylvania Pharmaceutical Assistance Contract for the Elderly (PACE) Pennsylvania | Claims data for PACE beneficiaries, 1984-1988; Medicare health services records; County-level demographic and health services resources databases | Human Resources Profile County Code from 1980 census data in Area Resource File (ARF: 10 levels depicting degree of rurality) | Age; gender; race; income; marital status; physicians, pharmacies, hospital beds, and nursing home beds per 1,000 population; outpatient physician visits; any physician visits, inpatient days, or any hospital day in past month | Moderate | Monthly claims(-); HR, U |

| Author, Year, Study Design | Characteristics of Study Population (Sample Size, Inclusion/Exclusion, Region of United States) | Data Source and Year(s) of Sampling (if applicable) Response rate (if applicable) | Definition of Urban/Rural | Covariates | Confidence Score* | Results** |
|---|---|---|---|---|---|---|
| Lillard, 1999[92] Cross-sectional | N = 910 Medicare enrollees ages 66 or older Excluded individuals covered by HMOs or institutionalized National | 1990 Elderly Health Supplement to the Panel Study of Income Dynamics (PSID), a nationally representative telephone/mail survey Response rate: 99% (telephone survey); 74%(mail survey) | Area Resource File (Department of Health and Human Services) | Age, gender, race, marital status, education, income, current health status, insurance status | Low | Twelve-month medication use: (-) Prescription cost (+); U>R |
| Mueller, 2004[93] Cross-sectional | N = 32,465,895 Noninstitutionalized Medicare beneficiaries 65 or older National | 1997 Medicare Current Beneficiary Survey; 1996 Medical Expenditure Panel Survey | Rural: any place of residence not in a Metropolitan Statistical Area (MSA) | Insurance status | Low;" Moderate | Total drug expenditures (-) Prescriptions filled (+); R>Uninsured U Prescriptions filled (+): Insured R>insured U |
| Rogowski, 1997[95] Cross-sectional | N = 996 Noninstitutionalized Medicare enrollees ages 66 or older National | Panel Study of Income Dynamics (PSID), 1990 Response rate: 99% (telephone survey); 74% (mail survey) | Rural: any place of residence not in a MSA | Age, education, gender, race, marital status, income, insurance status, health status | Low | Percentage of family income spent on medications (-) |
| Xu, 2003[94] Cross-sectional | N = 3,498 Noninstitutionalized elderly West Texas | Telephone survey, 2000 Response rate: 71% (phase 1); 89.3% (phase 2); 53.2% (both phase 1 and 2) | Urban (counties in MSA) Rural (counties outside MSA or population < 50,000) Frontier (counties with < 7 people/ square mile) | Race, age, gender, employment, income, insurance, usual source of care, physical and mental health-related quality of life, several health beliefs | Low | Odds of prescription drug use (-) R,U; (+) U>F Usual pharmacy (-) R,U; (+) U>F e |

*See Methods section for explanation

**U=Urban; R=Rural; HR=Highly rural; F=Frontier; (+)=difference statistically significant; (-)=difference not statistically significant

Rural vs. Urban Ambulatory Health Care: A Systematic Review

Evidence-based Synthesis Program

## Appendix C, Table 10. Medical Procedures and Diagnostic Tests

| Author, Year, Study Design | Characteristics of Study Population (Sample Size, Inclusion/Exclusion, Region of United States) | Data Source and Year(s) of Sampling (if applicable) Response rate (if applicable) | Definition of Urban/Rural | Covariates | Confidence Score* | Results** |
|---|---|---|---|---|---|---|
| Escarce et al., 1993[97]<br><br>Cross-sectional | N = 1,204,022<br><br>Inclusion: Medicare enrollees 65+ years<br><br>Exclusion: end-stage renal disease, covered by an HMO<br><br>National | Health Care Finance Administration (HCFA) Medicare Part B Annual Data Beneficiary File, 1986<br><br>HCFA Health Insurance Skeleton Eligibility Write-off File, 1986 | Rural: living in a nonmetropolitan county<br><br>Urban: living in a metropolitan county | Age, gender | Low | Rurality and race interaction (+); white-black relative risks for services were higher in rural areas for 12 of 32 studied services (including 8 of 14 outpatient services) |
| Miller et al., 1995[96]<br><br>Cross-sectional | N = 31,100,000<br><br>Medicare Part B beneficiaries<br><br>Excluded those enrolled in HMOs<br><br>National | Medicare Part B Annual Data File, 1990<br><br>Health Insurance Eligibility Write-off File, 1990 | Rural areas are the non-MSA areas of states. Urban areas are subdivided into small MSAs (less than 250,000 inhabitants), large MSAs (250,000 to 3 million), and very large MSAs (3 million or more). | Age, race, gender | Low | Physician utilization (+); R<U (particularly consultations, psychiatric visits, emergency department visits, imaging services, and laboratory tests) |

*See Methods section for explanation

**U=Urban; R=Rural; (+)=difference statistically significant; (–)=difference not statistically significant

Rural vs. Urban Ambulatory Health Care: A Systematic Review

Evidence-based Synthesis Program

## Appendix C, Table 11. Medical Appointments with Providers

| Author, Year, Study Design | Characteristics of Study Population (Sample Size, Inclusion/Exclusion, Region of United States) | Data Source and Year(s) of Sampling (if applicable) Response rate (if applicable) | Definition of Urban/Rural | Covariates | Confidence Score* | Results** |
|---|---|---|---|---|---|---|
| Blazer, 1995[98] Cross-sectional | N = 4,162 (4,001 respondents) Inclusion: ages 65+ years; resident of 1 of 5 counties 1 urban and 4 rural counties in North Carolina | Duke Established Populations for Epidemiologic Studies of the Elderly, 1986-1987 Response rate: 80% | US Bureau of the Census: rural is county with fewer than 2,500 inhabitants Also classified counties as rural or urban | Race/ethnicity, self-rated health, the health index, age, gender, education, marital status, employment status, income, Medicare coverage, Medicaid coverage, private insurance | Low/ Moderate | Ambulatory care visits (-) |
| Fortney, 2002[105] Cross-sectional | N = 355,452 Inclusion: primary care patients treated at 38 Community-Based Outpatient Clinics (CBOCs) or 32 parent VA Medical Centers (VAMCs) CBOCs and VAMCs from 16 Veterans Integrated Services Networks (VISNs) | Austin Automatic Center (AAC) outpatient file, 1995-1998 | Comparisons focused on CBOCs vs. VAMCs | Age, gender, marital status, ethnicity, service-connected, percent service connected, VA service use in prior year | Moderate | Primary care encounters (+): CBOC>VAMC Specialty care encounters (+): CBOC<VAMC Number of days to follow-up care for hospitalization or inpatient psychiatric treatment (-) |
| Glover, 2004[100] Cross-sectional | N = 50,993 (9,778 or 19% rural) Inclusion: ages 18-64 Nationwide | National Health Interview Surveys, 1999-2000 Response: 81% (1999) and 83% (2000) | Urban: Metropolitan Statistical Area Rural: Non-MSA | Race/ethnicity, gender, age, region of residence, interview language, limitations in activities, self-reported health status, education, employment, family size, income, marital status, insurance | Moderate | Health care use in past 12 months (-) (within urban and rural, minorities less likely to have visit (+)) |
| Himes & Rutrough, 1994[101] Cross-sectional | N = 11,101 Inclusion: non-institutionalized persons ages 65 and older Nationwide | National Health Interview Survey (Supplement on Aging), 1984 | Four categories: Metropolitan central city residents (within SMSAs); metropolitan noncentral city residents; nonmetropolitan nonfarm residents (outside SMSA); nonmetropolitan farm residents | Age, gender, ethnicity, marital status, education, health status, limitations in activities of daily living, living arrangement, poverty, region of U.S., bed disability days | Moderate | Physician visit in past year (+): non-metro<metro |

91

Rural vs. Urban Ambulatory Health Care: A Systematic Review

Evidence-based Synthesis Program

| Author, Year, Study Design | Characteristics of Study Population (Sample Size, Inclusion/Exclusion, Region of United States) | Data Source and Year(s) of Sampling (if applicable) Response rate (if applicable) | Definition of Urban/Rural | Covariates | Confidence Score* | Results** |
|---|---|---|---|---|---|---|
| Larson & Fleishman, 2003[102] Cross-sectional | N = 14,997 Inclusion: persons 18+ in second round interviews Exclusion: missing data for the independent variables, or died, became institutionalized, or moved out of the country in 1996 Nationwide | Medical Expenditure Panel Survey, 1996 | Nine-category Urban Influence Codes: Large MSA with 1million or more; small MSA with less than 1 million; adjacent large MSA with city of 10K or more; adjacent large MSA with city less than 10K; adjacent small MSA with city of 10K or more; adjacent small MSA with city less than 10K; not adjacent with city of 10K or more; not adjacent with city between 2.5-10K; non-adjacent with no town more than 2.5K | Gender, ethnicity, education, age, insurance, family income, self-reported health, priority condition, limitations in activities of daily living or instrumental activities of daily living, physician availability, region, has usual source of care | Moderate | Any ambulatory care visit (+); adjacent large MSA (with city <10k or > 10k) < MSA with ≥ 1million Any ambulatory care visit (-): most rural vs. most urban Number of ambulatory care visits (+): most rural < large MSA |
| Maciejewski, 2007[104] Cross-sectional | N = 63,478 Inclusion: primary care patients treated at one of 108 Community-Based Outpatient Clinics (CBOCs) and/or one of 72 parent VA Medical Centers (VAMCs) | VA FY2000 Outpatient Care File; VA FY2000 Patient Treatment File; VA FY2000 and FY2001 Decision Support System Outpatient and Inpatient National Extracts | Compared VAMC patients, CBOC patients, and crossover patients | Age, gender, race, marital status, eligibility for free care, service-related disability, DCG risk score, distance to usual source of care | High | Primary care visits (+); CBOC>VAMC Specialty care visits (+); CBOC<VAMC Total outpatient expenditures (+); CBOC<VAMC |
| McConnel & Zetzman, 1993[99] Cohort | N = 3,350 Inclusion: individuals 55 and older Exclusion: died, moved, could not be re-interviewed, or had missing data on relevant variables Nationwide | National Center for Health Statistics' Longitudinal Study of Aging, 1984-1986 Area Resource File, 1987 | U.S. Department of Agriculture (1989) 10-level County Adjacency Codes to create three categories: major urban (MSA counties), less urban (non-MSA counties with towns larger than 2.5K), and rural (non-MSA counties with towns with fewer than 2.5K) | Age, gender, ethnicity, living arrangement, social contact, education, prior service use, Medicaid eligibility, limitations in activities of daily living, health status, chronic conditions, and availability of hospital beds, physicians, and nursing home beds. | Low | Use of physician services (-) |

Rural vs. Urban Ambulatory Health Care: A Systematic Review

Evidence-based Synthesis Program

| Author, Year, Study Design | Characteristics of Study Population (Sample Size, Inclusion/Exclusion, Region of United States) | Data Source and Year(s) of Sampling (if applicable) Response rate (if applicable) | Definition of Urban/Rural | Covariates | Confidence Score* | Results** |
|---|---|---|---|---|---|---|
| Mueller, 1998[103]<br><br>Cross-sectional | N = 112,246<br><br>Inclusion: respondents under 65<br><br>Nationwide | National Health Interview Survey, 1992<br><br>Response rate: 95.7% | Urban: central or noncentral cities located within a MSA<br><br>Rural: outside a MSA, either on a farm or not | Age, gender, self-reported health status, presence of acute or chronic health problems, ethnicity, family size, education, insurance status, income, region of country | Moderate | Physician visit in past 12 months:<br><br>(+); any R<U White (except R African American) |
| Saag et al., 1998[29]<br><br>Cross-sectional | N = 787<br><br>Inclusion: home-dwelling elderly (age > 65 years), ≥ 1 of the indicator conditions, resident of state's 12 most rural and 10 most urban counties<br><br>Iowa | Population based phone survey evaluating six common chronic indicator conditions (arthritis, hypertension, cardiac disease, diabetes mellitus, peptic ulcer disease, and chronic obstructive pulmonary disease)<br><br>Response: 57% | U.S. Department of Agriculture continuum codes.<br><br>Urban: metro areas with > 250,000 residents<br><br>Rural: <2,500 residents in a single incorporated place and not adjacent to metro areas | Age, gender, education beyond high school, living on a farm, alcohol use, smoking in the past, medical advice needed in the past year, supplemental private insurance, medication coverage, Medicaid, VA clinic in the past year, Distance from physician, congregate meals, Use of Meals on Wheels, Homemaker service | Low | Number of physician visits (-) |
| Weeks et al., 2005[8]<br><br>Cohort | N = 67,985 (1997); 51,899 (1998); 56,833 (1999)<br><br>Inclusion: male veterans 65 years or older and enrolled in Medicare fee-for-service plans<br><br>New England | VHA's Patient Treatment File and Outpatient Clinic File, 1995-1999<br><br>Medicare Denominator, 100% MEDPAR, Outpatient, and Physician Supply files, 1997-1999 | Department of Agriculture Rural/Urban Commuting Area (RUCA) Code; grouped into urban (RUCA codes 1-6) and rural (RUCA codes 7-10) | Age, gender, living in the northern or southern states of New England, number of VHA and Medicare inpatient admissions | Moderate | Primary, specialist, and mental health visits (+); R<U (across all three study years ) |

*See Methods section for explanation

**U=Urban; R=Rural; HR=Highly rural; F=Frontier; (+)=difference statistically significant; (-)=difference not statistically significant

93

## Appendix C, Table 12. Usual Source of Care

| Author, Year, Study Design | Study Population (Sample Size, Inclusion/Exclusion, Region/Nationwide) | Data Source, Year(s) (if applicable) Response Rate (if applicable) | Definition of Urban/ Rural | Covariates | Confidence Score* | Results** |
|---|---|---|---|---|---|---|
| Meza, 2006[106] Cross-sectional | N = 3,871 Inclusion: Department of Defense beneficiaries, active duty, uniformed services Nationwide | Health Care Survey of DoD Beneficiearies (HCSDB) – mailed survey 2002 Response: 29% | US Census Bureau – metropolitan (metro), adjacent to metropolitan (adj), or nonadjacent (non adj) | Age, service category, marital status, self-reported health status, race, rank, gender, utilization, years in health plan, health plan, indicator of other health plan | Low | Rating of health plan, rating of health care, getting care quickly(+); Adj or non-adj> Metro  Getting needed care (+); Metro>Adj or non-adj |
| Blazer, 1995[98] Cross-sectional | N = 4,162 (2,152 or 47% rural); 4001 with complete data Inclusion: >65 yrs, resident of 1 urban or 4 rural counties North Carolina | Stratified (race & residence) random sample-Duke Established Populations for Epidemiologic Study of the Elderly survey, 1986-87 Response: 80% | US Bureau of the Census Rural: fewer than 2,500 inhabitants Also classified counties as rural or urban | Race/ethnicity, self-rated health, health index, age, gender, education, marital status, employment, income, Medicare and Medicaid coverage, private insurance | Low/ Moderate | Usual source of care (-) Usually sees same provider(+); R>U  Put off care due to not knowing where to go (-)  Put off care due to transportation difficulties (-)  Put off care due to cost (+); R>U |
| Borders, 2004[107] Cross-sectional | N = 2,097 Inclusion: community dwelling, age ≥65, Hispanic or non-Hispanic white West Texas | Telephone survey Response: 53% | Rural: county with fewer than 50,000 persons Frontier: county with fewer than 50,000 persons and fewer than 7 persons/mi² | Age, gender, ethnicity, marital status, education, economic factors, insurance, chronic conditions | Low/ Moderate | Always/usually see personal doctor/nurse (-)  Always/usually able to obtain care without a long wait (-) |
| Glover, 2004[100] Cross-sectional | N = 50,993 (9,778 or 19% rural) Inclusion: ages 18-64 Nationwide | National Health Interview Surveys, 1999-2000 Response: 81% (1999) and 83% (2000) | Rural: any place of residence not in a Metropolitan Statistical Area | Race/ethnicity, gender, age, interview language, region of residence, limitation of activities, self-reported health status, education, employment, family size, income, marital status, insurance | Low/ Moderate | Usual source of care (-) (in rural and urban areas Hispanic adults less likely than white adults to have usual source of care)  Health care use in past 12 months (-) |

| Author, Year, Study Design | Study Population (Sample Size, Inclusion/Exclusion, Region/Nationwide) | Data Source, Year(s) (if applicable) Response Rate (if applicable) | Definition of Urban/ Rural | Covariates | Confidence Score* | Results** |
|---|---|---|---|---|---|---|
| Koopman, 2006[48]<br><br>Cross-sectional | N = 947<br><br>Inclusion: US civilian, ≥20 years, non-institutionalized, participated in NHANES III: household adult, examination, and laboratory data files<br><br>Exclusion: did not participate in all three parts of the survey<br><br>Nationwide | Third National Health and Nutrition Examination Survey (NHANES III) 1988-1994 | Urban: MSA<br><br>Rural: Non-MSA | Gender, age, BMI, perceived health status, income, insurance status, education, usual place of care, # times seeing physician in past year, duration of diabetes | Moderate | Usual source of care (+); U Hispanic<R Hispanic, R White, U White#<br><br>#Unadjusted analysis |
| Larson, 2003[102]<br><br>Cross-sectional | N = 15,518 for geographic variation<br><br>N = 14,997 for regression<br><br>Inclusion: non-institutionalized, civilian, age 18 and older<br><br>Nationwide | Medical Expenditures Panel Survey (MEPS), 1996<br><br>Area Resource File (ARF) with Urban Influence Codes (UIC) | UICs by county – large (pop'l >1 million) or small metropolitan areas; non-metropolitan areas distinguished by adjacency and pop'l of largest city (>10,000) | Gender, ethnicity, education, age, insurance, family income, self-reported health, priority condition, limitations in activities of daily living or instrumental activities of daily living, physician availability, region, usual source of care | Moderate | Usual source of care (+); most R>most U (adj. to large MSA with city <10,000 also greater than most urban) |
| Rohrer, 2004[18]<br><br>Cross-sectional | N = 3,689 (1,983 or 54% rural)<br><br>N,=3,680 for usual source of care outcome<br><br>Inclusion: ages 65 and older<br><br>West Texas | Texas Tech 5000 telephone survey, Sept.-Dec. 2000<br><br>Response: 57% | Rural: county with population less than 50,000 | Age, gender, ethnicity, resides in continuing care, health limitations, specific diagnoses, education, income, marital status, medical skepticism, religiousness, insurance status, employment, home ownership | Low | Personal doctor or nurse (-)<br><br>Usual place to go for care (-) |

*See Methods section for explanation

**U=Urban; R=Rural; (+)=difference statistically significant; (-)=difference not statistically significant

95

Rural vs. Urban Ambulatory Health Care: A Systematic Review

Evidence-based Synthesis Program

## Appendix C, Table 13. Provider Availability and Expertise

| Author, Year, Study Design | Study Population (Sample Size, Inclusion/Exclusion, Region/Nationwide) | Data Source, Year(s) (if applicable) Response Rate (if applicable) | Definition of Urban/Rural | Covariates | Confidence Score* | Results** |
|---|---|---|---|---|---|---|
| Baldwin, 1999[117] Cross-sectional | N = 4,003 physicians (619 or 15.5% rural); 382,776 patients of those physicians<br><br>Inclusion: physicians practicing in either rural or urban areas (not both); specialties with at least 10 physicians submitting claims in rural and urban locations; Medicare beneficiaries (65 and older)<br><br>Washington | Medicare Part B file (billed services), 1994<br><br>Health Care Financing Administration (HCFA) provider directory<br><br>Medicare beneficiary file | Rural Health Service Areas defined as physician practice addresses with ZIP codes closer to rural hospital than urban hospital | None | Low/Moderate | Family physicians most likely to practice in rural area (25%), psychiatrists (5%), cardiologists (6%), gastroenterologist (8%) least likely_#<br><br>Family physician age (+); R>U#<br><br>Patients/physician (+); R>U#<br><br>Outpatient visits/physician (+); R>U#<br><br>Diagnostic scope of practice similar except: urban general surgeons >CV disorders; rural general surgeons >GI disorders and urban obstetrician-gynecologists >care for menopausal symptoms; rural obstetrician-gynecologists >diagnoses outside specialty#<br><br>Procedure rates (+); R>U for family practice, internal medicine, general surgery#<br>#Unadjusted analysis |
| Biola, 2009[111] Cross-sectional | N = 4,879 from 150 rural counties<br><br>Inclusion: English- or Spanish-speaking, age ≥18, lived in community for previous 12 months (1 person selected from each household reached)<br><br>Southeast (AL, AK, GA, LA, MS, SC, TX, WV) | Telephone survey 2002-2003; this report focused on question: How much do you agree with the statement: 'I feel there are enough doctors in my community?'<br><br>Response: 51% | Not reported<br><br>NOTE: counties selected by project leaders; typically higher poverty and unemployment rates, larger racial-ethnic minority proportions, and higher infant mortality rates than other rural counties in the state | Age, gender, race, education, children <18 years, self-reported health, health insurance status, travel time to care, problem with cost of care, ease of getting appointment, role of physician care, number of visits in past year, satisfaction with care, confidence in doctor's abilities, county characteristics | Low | Not enough physicians (+):<br><br>a. areas with fewer physicians/pop'l > areas with more physicians/pop'l<br><br>b. travel time to care more than 30 min > travel time to care less than 30 min |

| Author, Year, Study Design | Study Population (Sample Size, Inclusion/Exclusion, Region/Nationwide) | Data Source, Year(s) (if applicable) Response Rate (if applicable) | Definition of Urban/Rural | Covariates | Confidence Score* | Results** |
|---|---|---|---|---|---|---|
| Brown B, 2009[109] Cross-sectional | N = 264 (132 self-reported rural) Primary care physician assistants (PAs) Nationwide | Web-based survey, 2008 (10 case-scenarios) Response: 49% responded; 44% analyzed | Respondents self-reported rural or urban | None | Low | Mean score on 10 question case-scenario quiz (+); R>U# PAs reporting they diagnose and treat 50-100% of skin complaints (+); R>U# Cases referred to specialist per week (-)# #Unadjusted analysis |
| Everett, 2009[113] Cross-sectional | N = 6,803 (887 or 13% non-metropolitan) Inclusion: graduated from high school in Wisconsin in 1957 or one of their siblings; stated they had usual source of care in 2004-05; specified a physician assistant (PA), nurse practitioner (NP), or physician (MD) with primary care specialty as usual provider Wisconsin | Wisconsin Longitudinal Study (WLS) - telephone and mail survey 1993-94 for perceived health, 2004-05 survey defined sample and all other variables Response: 80% for graduates, 78% for siblings (telephone); 88% for graduates and 81% for siblings (mailed survey to those who did telephone interview) | Office of Management and Budget (metropolitan, micropolitan, or nonmetropolitan) | Age, gender, marital status, education, insurance, personality traits, income, insurance, perceived health, number of diagnoses | Low/ Moderate | 306 (4.5%) use PA/NPs as usual source of care# PA/NP as usual source of care (+); non-metro>metro, non-metro>micro #Unadjusted analysis |
| Ferrer, 2007[110] Cross-sectional | N = 34,403 Inclusion: all ages, non-institutionalized, able to link household component with office and outpatient facility face-to-face visits Nationwide | MEPS, 2004 plus information from relevant clinicians Response (to MEPS): 64% | Metropolitan Statistical Area (MSA) = urban, non-MSA = rural | Age, gender, income, insurance, race/ethnicity | Low/ Moderate | Odds of visiting family physician, nurse practitioner, and physician assistant (+); non-MSA>MSA Odds of visiting general internist or non-surgical specialist (+); non-MSA<MSA |

Rural vs. Urban Ambulatory Health Care: A Systematic Review

Evidence-based Synthesis Program

| Author, Year, Study Design | Study Population (Sample Size, Inclusion/Exclusion, Region/Nationwide) | Data Source, Year(s) (if applicable) Response Rate (if applicable) | Definition of Urban/Rural | Covariates | Confidence Score* | Results** |
|---|---|---|---|---|---|---|
| Grumbach, 2003[112] Cross-sectional | N = 33,673 clinicians (28,053 California [CA], 5,620 Washington [WA]) Inclusion: active in patient care, no longer in training, primary self-reported specialty of family/general practice, internal medicine, pediatrics, obstetrics/gynecology California, Washington | AMA Physician Masterfile plus WA licensing board information and contacts with rural physicians (physician data) Mailed survey (non-physician data) Response: 64% (CA); 67% NPs in WA, 86% PAs in WA | CA: Medical Service Study Areas (MSSA); rural – population density <250 residents/mi$^2$ with no city of ≥50,000 WA: Rural Health Service Areas (HSA) and urban public health department zones; rural – core city or town non MSA or in MSA but >30 min from population base of ≥10,000 Census data | Clinician age, gender, and race/ethnicity | Low | 22% of Physician Assistants in CA practice in rural area; 28% in WA# Odds of practicing in rural areas: (+) family physicians, nurse practitioners, and physician assistants more likely relative to obstetricians/gynecologists (+) Asian, African Americans, Latinos (CA only) less likely (+) females less likely #Unadjusted analysis |
| Gunderson, 2006[115] Cross-sectional | N = 539 physicians who practiced in rural Florida Inclusion: physicians who self-report treating elderly (primary care, psychiatry, surgery, specialists) Florida | Mailed survey 2003 Response: 43% | Rural: one of 33 designated rural counties in Florida, practicing in rural areas of nonrural counties by Rural Commuting Area codes, or Health Resources and Services Administration list of rural ZIP codes | None | Low | 55% reported decreased or eliminated patient services in past year including mental health, (35%), vaccine administration (29%), office-based surgeries (40%), Pap smears (24%), x-rays (24%), endoscopies (43%), and electrocardiograms (11%)# Physicians in practice where ≥65% of patients were Medicare patients were more likely to reduce or eliminate services compared to those with <28.5% Medicare patients# #Unadjusted analysis |
| Jones, 2008[114] Cross-sectional | N = 254 counties Inclusion: all counties in Texas Texas | Texas Medical Board US Census Bureau, 2007 | Frontier - ≤6 people per 2.6 km$^2$ | None | High | 17 counties had no licensed doctors or physician assistants# Statewide: 1 physician assistant per 13.6 physicians Frontier counties: 1 physician assistant per 2.3 physicians# #Unadjusted analysis |

**Rural vs. Urban Ambulatory Health Care: A Systematic Review**

| Author, Year, Study Design | Study Population (Sample Size, Inclusion/Exclusion, Region/Nationwide) | Data Source, Year(s) (if applicable) Response Rate (if applicable) | Definition of Urban/Rural | Covariates | Confidence Score* | Results** |
|---|---|---|---|---|---|---|
| Laditka 2009[28] Cross-sectional | Inclusion: all US counties Nationwide | Area Resource File, 2002 | Urban Influence Codes, 2003 | None | High | Mean primary care physician supply (per 10,000 population): *Metropolitan:* 17.8 (large), 16.9 (small) *Micropolitan:* 12.3 (adj. to large metro), 13.1 (adj. to small metro) *Rural:* 7.1 (adj.t o small metro), 7.2 (adj. to micro), 9.2 (not adj. to metro or micro)# #Unadjusted analysis |
| Menachemi, 2006[116] Cross-sectional | N = 308 family physicians (176 rural, 132 urban) Florida | Mailed survey Response: 42% | Rural: one of 33 designated rural counties in Florida, practicing in rural areas of nonrural counties by Rural Urban Commuting Area codes, or Health Resources and Services Administration list of rural ZIP codes | None | Low | Overall, 60% reported delivery of patient services decreased or eliminated in past year# Types of services decreased or eliminated (-) (except for office-based surgeries)# #Unadjusted analysis |
| Strickland, 1998[118] Cross-sectional | N = 1,118 providers (1,079 with ZIP codes) Inclusion: nurse practitioners (NP), certified nurse midwives (CNM), physician assistants (PA) residing or practicing in Georgia Georgia | Mailed survey, 1994 Response: 62% | Metropolitan Statistical Area (MSA) = urban, non-MSA = rural | None | Low/ Moderate | NPs (n=554, 31% rural): older, fewer with bachelor's degree, fewer specialty credentials, more years in health care, more solo and clinic practice settings, fewer insured patients (+); R vs. U# CNMs (n=73, 29% rural): fewer specialty credentials, more hours per week, more patients per hour (+); R vs. U# PAs (n=452, 18% rural): older, fewer with bachelor's degree, more years in health care and years as PA, more patients each hour, more clinic practice settings, fewer insured patients (+); R vs. U# #Unadjusted analysis |

Rural vs. Urban Ambulatory Health Care: A Systematic Review

Evidence-based Synthesis Program

| Author, Year, Study Design | Study Population (Sample Size, Inclusion/Exclusion, Region/Nationwide) | Data Source, Year(s) (if applicable) Response Rate (if applicable) | Definition of Urban/Rural | Covariates | Confidence Score* | Results** |
|---|---|---|---|---|---|---|
| Wilson, 2009[66]<br><br>Cross-sectional | N = 1,427 counties or county sets (contiguous, single state sets of counties merged to achieve population >50,000)<br><br>Inclusion: all US counties or county sets except Alaska, Hawaii, and 12 cities with changes in county definitions between 1980 and 2000<br><br>Nationwide | Numbers of rehabilitation therapists (physical [PT] or occupational [OT] therapists, speech-language pathologists [SLP]) from 1980 and 1990 ARF and 2000 EEO<br><br>Health Professional Shortage Area Data | US Office of Management and Budget (OMB) – metropolitan (metro): central county with ≥1 urbanized area and outlying counties economically tied to core county | None | Moderate/ High | PTs, OTs, or SLPs per 100,000 residents (NR); U>R[#]<br><br>PTs, OTs, or SLPs per 100,000 residents (NR); Non-shortage area > partial or total shortage area[#] |

*See Methods section for explanation

**U=Urban; R=Rural; (+)=difference statistically significant; (-)=difference not statistically significant